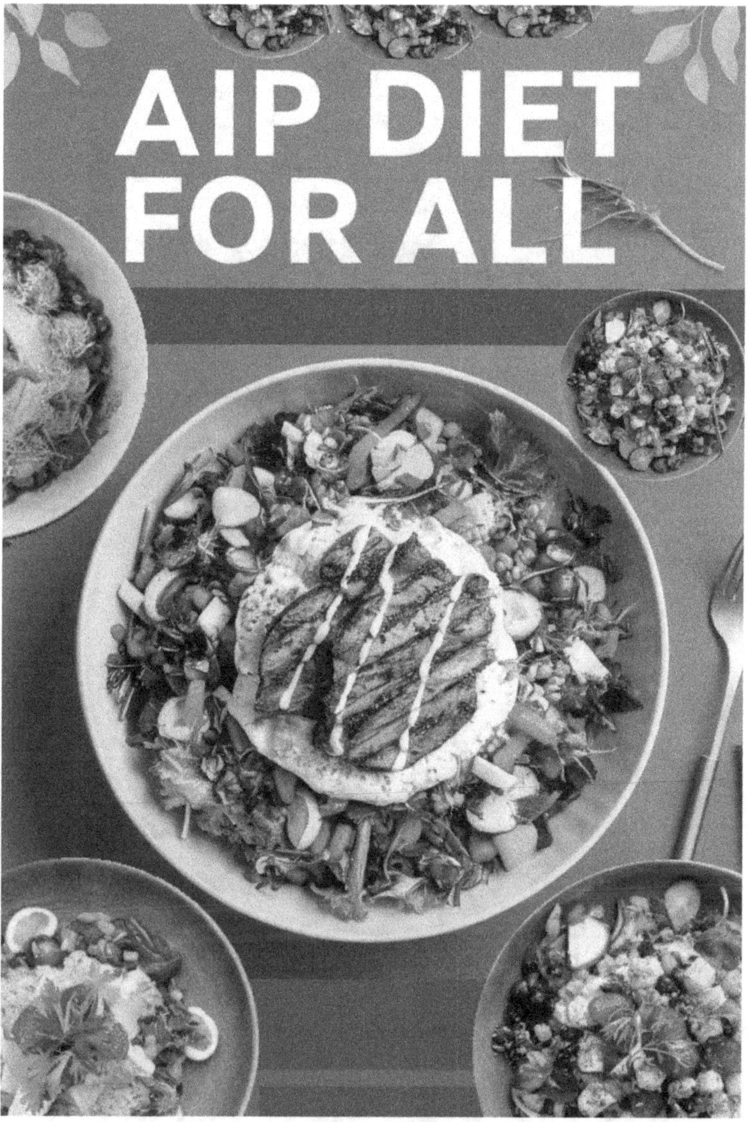

AIP DIET FOR ALL

AIP DIET COOKBOOK

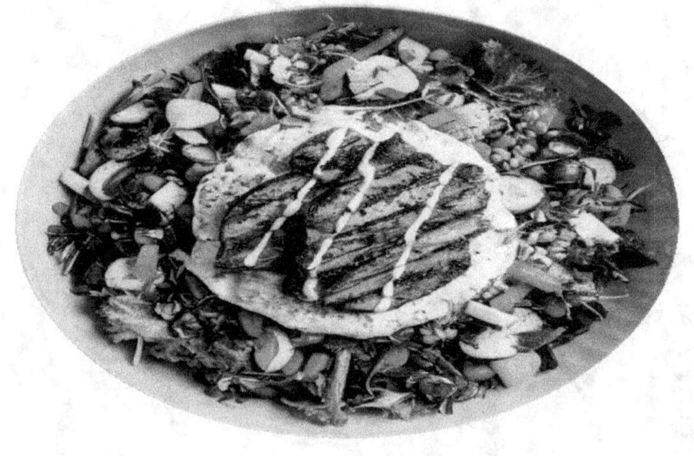

Guide to Quick, Easy, and Delicious Low-Carb Recipes for a Healthy and Vibrant Life

---

Rosell L Sophe

WITH A 30 DAYS MEAL PLANNER

Thank you for purchasing the Kindle version of my book! For a more comprehensive experience, consider upgrading to the paperback edition, which includes a bonus meal planner to help you stay on track with your goals.

GRATITUDE SPEECH:

Thank you all for coming out tonight to celebrate the launch of my book. Writing it has been a dream come true, but a book needs readers to complete it. I'm grateful to each and every one of you who purchased a copy. Your support means so much.

Special thanks to my family for your belief in me. To the booksellers for sharing my work, and most of all to readers for giving this book a chance and hopefully finding something of value within.

This experience has been enriched by your enthusiasm. Thank you for being part of this journey. Here's to many more stories to come. Cheers to you all!

Forward

I am thrilled to introduce this new book to readers. As an author, nothing is more rewarding than sharing ideas, stories and lessons that may strike a chord or provide fresh perspectives.

When I first started writing, my goal was simple – to explore concepts close to my heart and experience in the hope it may resonate with others. I had no idea the journey would lead here, but I am beyond grateful for the opportunity.

Within these pages you'll find discussions, reflections and case studies meant to both entertain and inspire. Some topics may challenge conventional thinking while others aim to empower. Above all, my aim has been to start meaningful dialog and give voice to insightful views.

For anyone who picks up this book, I hope you find nuggets of wisdom to ponder or sparks of motivation to pursue your dreams.

Know that every reader helps fuel my passion for using this craft to spread messages of hope.

It is with profound appreciation that I offer my work to you. Enjoy the journey that unfolds on these pages. My wish is that it enriches your mind, lifts your spirit and stays with you long after you've closed the cover.

Thank you for taking this journey with me. I hope to welcome you along with many more to come.

[ROSELL L SOPHE]

Table of Contents

Introduction to the Autoimmune Protocol (AIP) Diet

The Autoimmune Protocol, commonly known as the AIP diet, is an eliminative diet designed to help reduce inflammation and support healing in people with autoimmune diseases.

This article will provide an overview of the AIP diet, including its basic principles and goals. It will also introduce some common autoimmune conditions that the AIP diet aims to address.

What is the AIP Diet?

The Autoimmune Protocol (AIP) is an elimination diet that works to address chronic, low-grade systemic inflammation in the body.

This inflammation is thought to play a role in the development and worsening of autoimmune diseases. By removing certain food triggers from the diet, the goal of AIP is to reduce inflammation and support the body's natural healing processes.

The AIP diet was developed based on the identification of common food sensitivities and allergies seen in autoimmune patients. Some of the most problematic foods include:

- Grains (wheat, barley, rye, etc.)
- Legumes
- Dairy
- Eggs
- Nightshade vegetables (tomatoes, peppers, potatoes, eggplant)
- Added sugars
- Alcohol
- Coffee/black tea

By eliminating these potential triggers, the diet aims to give the gut lining a chance to heal.

It is believed that compromised gut barrier function may allow improperly digested food proteins and microbes to enter the bloodstream, promoting an autoimmune response.

In addition to food elimination, the AIP diet emphasizes the inclusion of nutrient-dense whole foods like meat, seafood, vegetables, fruits, nuts and healthy fats.

Fermented and cultured foods are also encouraged to support healthy gut bacteria balance.

The overall goal is to provide the body with nutrients for natural healing while reducing external stressors that may be perpetuating chronic inflammation.

The AIP diet is intended to be followed for at least 30-90 days as an elimination phase. This allows symptoms and sensitivities to be identified.

Then, foods can slowly be reintroduced one at a time to determine individual tolerance levels.

Understanding Autoimmune Diseases

Autoimmune diseases develop when the immune system mistakenly attacks and damages healthy body tissues.

It's believed that a combination of genetic, environmental, and lifestyle factors can trigger autoimmunity in susceptible individuals. Some of the most common autoimmune conditions include:

Rheumatoid Arthritis (RA) - An inflammatory disorder that causes pain, swelling, stiffness and loss of function in the joints. It can affect the hands, feet, wrists, knees, ankles and elbows.

Multiple Sclerosis (MS) - A disease where the immune system eats away at the protective myelin sheath that covers nerve fibers in the central nervous system.

This damage disrupts communication between the brain and body and causes unpredictable symptoms.

Inflammatory Bowel Disease (IBD) - A group of conditions (chiefly ulcerative colitis and Crohn's disease) that cause chronic inflammation within the digestive tract.

Symptoms vary but may include abdominal pain, diarrhea, rectal bleeding, weight loss and fatigue.

Type 1 Diabetes - An autoimmune disease where the immune system destroys the insulin-producing beta cells within the pancreas. This does not allow for proper blood sugar regulation.

Hashimoto's Thyroiditis - An autoimmune disorder where the thyroid gland is attacked by antibodies, causing it to become inflamed and fail to produce adequate thyroid hormones. Common symptoms include fatigue, cold sensitivity, weight gain and constipation.

Psoriasis - A skin condition where the immune system speeds up the growth cycle of skin cells. This causes flaky, itchy patches of red raised skin to form on any part of the body including the scalp, elbows and knees.

Lupus - A chronic autoimmune disease that can affect many different body systems including the joints, skin, kidneys, blood cells, brain, heart and lungs. Common symptoms are joint pains, rash, headaches, fatigue, chest pain and hair loss.

Vitiligo - Characterized by loss of skin color in patches due to destruction of melanocytes (cells that give color to the skin). Patches of skin appear lighter or complete white depending on the extent of melanocyte loss.

Autoimmune diseases can have tremendous physical, mental and emotional impacts on quality of life. They often require lifelong medical management as currently there are no cures.

The AIP diet aims to control symptoms and support overall wellness through targeted nutrition and lifestyle strategies.

Principles of the AIP Diet

The core principles of the Autoimmune Protocol diet focus on reducing inflammation through food and lifestyle modifications. Here are the key points of an AIP approach:

Food Elimination - To reduce triggers, AIP involves elimination of common food allergens and sensitivities like grains, dairy, eggs, legumes, nightshades, added sugars and more for 30-90+ days.

Inclusion of Whole Foods - Emphasis is placed on eating nutrient-dense plant foods like fruits, vegetables, healthy fats, grass-fed/pasture-raised meats, seafood, nuts and seeds.

Gut Healing - Fermented foods, bone broth and adequate hydration support healthy gut microbiome balance. Probiotics may also be used but check individual tolerance.

Stress Management - Techniques like yoga, meditation, journalling and spending time outdoors help counter stress which can exacerbate autoimmune symptoms.

Toxin Avoidance - Exposure to chemicals, molds, pesticides and other environmental triggers should be limited where possible.

Supplementation - Targeted supplements may be used to address nutritional deficiencies and support healing based on individual needs and medical guidance.

Reintroduction - After 30-90 days, foods are slowly reintroduced one at a time over several weeks to help identify personal sensitivities and tolerance levels.

Consistency - Strict adherence is generally recommended for at least six months before significant improvements may be seen. Patience and lifestyle changes are key to long-term results.

The AIP protocol aims to halt further deterioration and support natural self-healing by reducing food-related triggers and promoting gut, immune and overall health through a multi-pronged approach. Individual results will vary based on diseases and commitment to the lifestyle.

Transitioning to AIP

Making the transition to the Autoimmune Protocol diet requires some preparation both practically and mentally. Here are some tips for getting started:

- Meal plan and grocery shop ahead of time to ensure availability of compliant whole foods. Stock up on basics.

- Read labels carefully as common allergens hide in many products. Switch over personal care products, supplements, medications as needed.

- Slowly use up non-compliant foods at home over 1-2 weeks or give to friends/family. Throw out openly. Deep clean kitchen.

- Mindset shifts from deprivation to empowerment through self-care. Track improvements for encouragement during challenge times.

- Prepare simple recipes in advance or on weekends for easy grab-and-go breakfasts/lunches. Cook extra for leftovers.

- Consider support from an AIP-friendly health coach, dietitian or community groups online for recipe ideas and accountability.

- Expect symptoms to potentially worsen initially as the body detoxifies ("healing crisis"). Stay hydrated and rest when needed.

- Be patient through the process. Significant health changes often require consistency over several months to understand full impact.

Starting the AIP diet may seem daunting but focusing on small, positive step-by-step actions to prepare the body and home makes it very manageable. Remember the long-term benefits of reducing inflammation and supporting natural healing.

Sample Meal Plan

Here is a sample weekly AIP menu to provide meal and snack ideas:

Breakfast:
- Eggs scrambled with veggies
- Fruit smoothie with nut butter
- Coconut yogurt parfait with berries
- Sweet potato hash

Lunch:
- Lettuce wraps with chicken, avocado, carrots

- Salmon salad
- Leftover soup in a thermos
- Roast beef and vegetable steamed

Dinner:
- Beef stir fry with broccoli and brown rice
- Baked fish with roasted root vegetables
- Chicken thighs with sauteed kale and mushrooms
- Turkey chili with cauliflower "rice"

Snacks:
- Hard boiled eggs
- Apple with almond butter
- Vegetables and hummus
- Roast chickpeas
- Beef or turkey jerky
- Gluten-free crackers with nut butter

Treats:
- Coconut milk pudding
- Chocolates made without top allergens
- Homemade chips (sweet potato, plantain etc)
- Fruit and nut bars

A balanced variety ensures adequate nutrients while keeping options simple and easy to prepare. Meal planning is important for long-term AIP success and compliance.

AIP Diet Benefits and Results

When followed strictly for several months, many people with autoimmune diseases see promising results from the AIP protocol. Some common reported benefits include:

- Reduced inflammation levels overall as measured by markers like ESR and CRP
- Decreased autoimmune disease symptoms and/or fewer flare ups
- Improvement in gut health issues like
- Improved gut health issues like IBS, Crohn's, ulcerative colitis
- Weight regulation and fat loss without calorie counting
- Better energy levels and sense of well-being
- Clearer thinking and improved mood
- Reduced joint pain or stiffness from conditions like RA, lupus

- Skin clear of eczema, psoriasis or other rashes flaring up
- Regrowth of pigment in areas affected by vitiligo
- Fewer neurological symptoms for MS or other autoimmune diseases
- Potential reversal or remission of some conditions over time

While results are gradual and individual, many see at least partial symptom relief within a few months on AIP if dietary and lifestyle triggers are largely addressed.

Conditions affecting quality of life the most tend to show the clearest improvements.

Following strict protocols long-term is generally needed for more chronic conditions to improve significantly.

People may also find that non-autoimmune health issues clear up on the AIP diet such as headaches, chronic infections, digestive complaints, insomnia, anxiety or fatigue of unknown causes.

This suggests broader anti-inflammatory benefits beyond just autoimmune conditions.

Managing stress, practicing self-care, drinking sufficient water daily and exercising also enhance outcomes when combined with the AIP nutrition plan.
The diet alone is insufficient without additional lifestyle modifications to curb inflammation at its root causes.

No one is guaranteed to achieve remission by following AIP alone depending on autoimmune disease severity and other individual factors.

But most experience at least some degree of relief from implementing its anti-inflammatory strategies consistently over several months.

For some, it provides the tools to gain control over symptoms and improve overall wellness quality day by day.

Common Autoimmune Conditions

Now that we've covered the basics of the AIP diet, let's explore some specific autoimmune diseases and conditions that it may help address:

Rheumatoid Arthritis

Rheumatoid arthritis (RA) is a chronic inflammatory disorder that causes pain, swelling and stiffness in the joints.

It can affect both small and large joints, including hands, wrists, knees, feet, elbows and shoulders. Some key aspects of RA:

- Affects around 1% of the general population, mostly women.
- Occurs when the immune system attacks joint tissues, causing inflammation.
- May lead to joint deformity, contractures and loss of mobility over time.
- Common symptoms include fatigue, low-grade fever, loss of appetite.

- Standard medical treatment involves disease-modifying anti-rheumatic drugs.

For RA patients, following the anti-inflammatory AIP diet has been shown to help relieve joint pain and stiffness.
Reducing dietary triggers of inflammation provides synergistic support with medications to better control symptoms and slow joint damage progression.

Inflammatory Bowel Disease

The two main types of inflammatory bowel disease (IBD) are Crohn's disease and ulcerative colitis.
IBD causes chronic gastrointestinal inflammation and uncomfortable symptoms:
- Crohn's can affect any part of the digestive tract with symptoms like diarrhea, abdominal pain, weight loss.
- Colitis only involves the large intestine with blood in stool as a main symptom.
- Combined these affect 1-2 million Americans and 10-15 per 100,000 worldwide.

- Conventional treatment includes biologics, immunosuppressants, corticosteroids.

For IBD, the AIP dietary approach has demonstrated benefits in inducing and maintaining remission of symptoms by addressing gut inflammation at its source. Several studies show promise in conjunction with drug therapy.

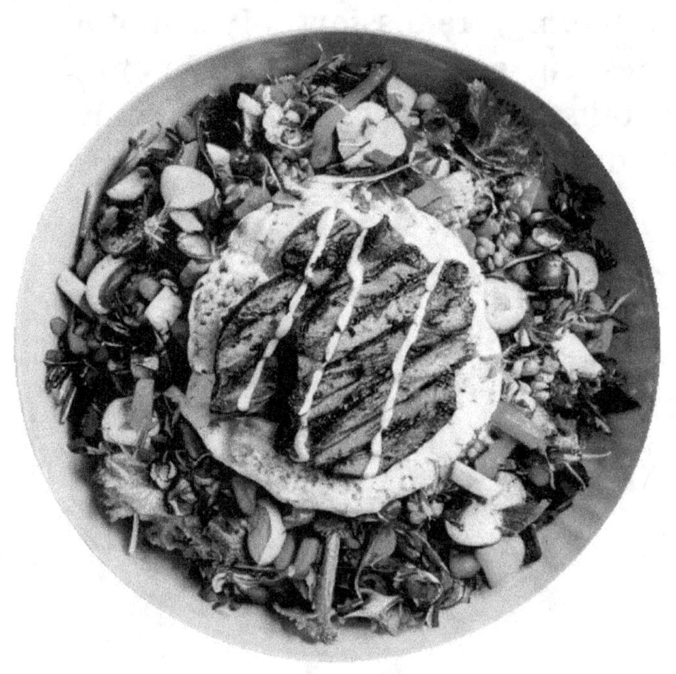

Chapter 1

The Science Behind the AIP Diet

While more research is still needed, there is growing scientific evidence that supports the mechanisms by which the AIP diet may help manage autoimmune conditions.

Gut-Immune Connection

The gut and immune system are deeply interconnected. Compromised intestinal barrier function allows undigested food particles, toxins, and microbes to enter the bloodstream, activating the immune system inappropriately.

This chronic low-grade inflammation has been linked to various autoimmune diseases.

Studies show that elimination of common food allergens from dairy, grains, legumes and nightshades can help repair the gut lining and reduce its permeability. This seals the barrier and prevents harmful compounds from triggering further immune reactions.

Microbiome Modulation

Imbalances in the gut microbiome composition are associated with heightened intestinal inflammation and systemic disease activity in autoimmunity.

The microbiome interacts strongly with the immune system through diet and metabolites produced.

Research indicates that elimination and anti-inflammatory aspects of the AIP diet such as fermented foods can beneficially reshape the microbiome over time.

This calms gut inflammation and related autoimmune symptoms. More diversity in gut bacteria is consistently seen in remission.

Lower Toxin Load

Refined foods, additives, pesticides and other environmental toxins place a large burden on the liver and immune system.

Toxic byproducts must be continuously processed and eliminated which induces oxidative stress.

Limiting toxic exposures and supporting detox pathways is an underappreciated element of the AIP approach.

Reducing overall toxic load through whole, pure foods may give the body energy to focus on self-repair instead of constant threat response.

Nutritional Support

Many autoimmune patients have underlying nutrient deficiencies that impair natural healing and detox abilities. The targeted inclusion of foods rich in vitamins A, C, D, E,

B12, magnesium, omega-3s and others addressed critical support gaps.

Providing building blocks to regenerate tissues and an anti-inflammatory nutrient profile empowers the body's natural restoration processes over the long-term following AIP guidelines.

Detox support from glutathione-boosting foods also helps remove cellular debris.

Personalized Protocol

Not all triggers equally impact everyone, so identification through elimination and reintroduction phases pinpoints the most reactive dietary elements specific to the individual. This personalized approach is very powerful.

Relevant food allergies and sensitivities are targeted accordingly versus a one-size-fits-all plan. Further customization based on genetic testing may offer even more precision, though cost can be prohibitive currently for many.

The science demonstrates several synergistic mechanisms by which the multi-faceted AIP diet supports natural resolution of autoimmunity through gut healing, microbiome balancing, lowered toxic burden and targeted nutrition. Further research continues to uncover valuable insights.

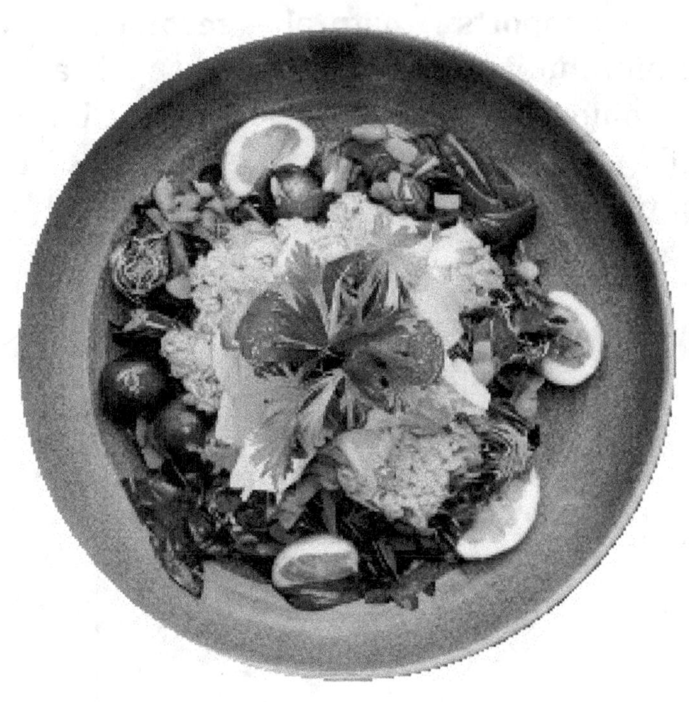

Chapter 2

Getting Started with the AIP Diet

Transitioning to the AIP way of eating does require some preparation. Here are some tips for getting your kitchen stocked and ready for AIP cooking:

Grocery Shopping List

- Make a shopping list of all the basic compliant foods you'll need like various meats, seafood, veggies, fruits, healthy fats.

- Look for brands and items certified gluten-free to avoid cross-contamination risks.

- Check labels carefully for hidden allergens like seeds/nuts in packaged goods.

- Stock up on pantry items like coconut flour, almond flour, nut butters, coconut aminos sauce, gelatin, bone broth.

- Buy compliant sweeteners like honey, maple syrup, dates for recipes.

Clearing Out the Pantry

- Go through all the cabinets and drawers, pulling out anything containing foods to eliminate like grains, legumes, sugar, coffee etc.

- Give away non-compliant foods to friends/family or dispose of open items properly so they're not a temptation.

- Check spice jars for non-pure ingredients like dairy, sugar, starch fillers. Replace as needed.

Kitchen Equipment

- Having basic equipment makes prep easier
- knives, cutting boards, pots/pans, baking dishes, mixing bowls, colander.

- Consider an instant read food thermometer for meats, an immersion blender for sauces.

- Procure supplies like parchment paper, aluminum foil, plastic wrap, ziplocks for food storage.

Food Prep Essentials

- Cooking in bulk and prepping ingredients ahead of time saves time and money.

- Some staples to have on hand include compliant oils, broths, fermented veggies, roasted veggies/meats, cooked eggs, nut flours.

- Buy in-season produce to enjoy variety while sticking to diet guidelines.

Cleaning Your Kitchen

- Do a thorough cleaning to remove any traces of banned foods.

- Consider natural, non-toxic cleaning products without dyes, perfumes or potential allergens.

A well-stocked kitchen makes following AIP sustainable long-term. With the right foundation, you'll be able to whip up healthy, delicious meals with ease.

Chapter 3

Key Components of the AIP Diet

In order to manage symptoms successfully, it's important to understand precisely which foods the AIP diet allows and avoids. Here are the foundational components:

Foods to Include

- Vegetables (except nightshades): All non-starchy veggies add nutrients, fiber and antioxidants.

- Healthy Fats: Olive oil, coconut oil, avocado, nuts/seeds in moderation. Fats provide energy and support cell functions.

- High-Quality Proteins: Grass-fed/pasture-raised meats, wild-caught fish, organic poultry, eggs from pastured hens.

- Fruits: Fresh and frozen fruit in moderation. Berries are ideal choices.

- Fermented & Cultured Foods: Unsweetened kefir, yogurt, kimchi, sauerkraut support beneficial gut bacteria.

- Bone Broth: Sip homemade broth for minerals, gelatin and healing properties.

- Herbs & Spices: Fresh spices add flavor without common allergens like garlic and onion.

Foods to Initially Avoid

- Grains: All types of wheat, barley, rye, oats, corn, rice, millet, quinoa, buckwheat and relatives.

- Legumes: Beans, peas, lentils and soy in all forms including edamame, tofu, tempeh, miso.

- Dairy: Milk, cheese, yogurt, butter, cream, ice cream, ghee, casein, whey.

- Eggs: Due to lectin content in whites and yolks.

- Nightshade Vegetables: Tomatoes, bell peppers, chili peppers, eggplant, white potatoes and relatives.

- Added Sugar: Refined cane sugar, brown sugar, honey, maple syrup, agave and artificial sweeteners.

- Alcohol: Beer, wine, liquor disrupt gut microbiome and liver function.

- Coffee/Black Tea: Caffeine is an inflammatory compound. Herbal tea is allowed.

Strict elimination, aside from reintroductions, is followed for a minimum of 30 days for dietary triggers to fully leave the system. Then individual tolerance can be assessed.

Sticking to these straightforward guidelines forms the underpinning of the AIP protocol for health restoration. Over time, a personalized way of eating will become clear as symptoms guide reintroductions.

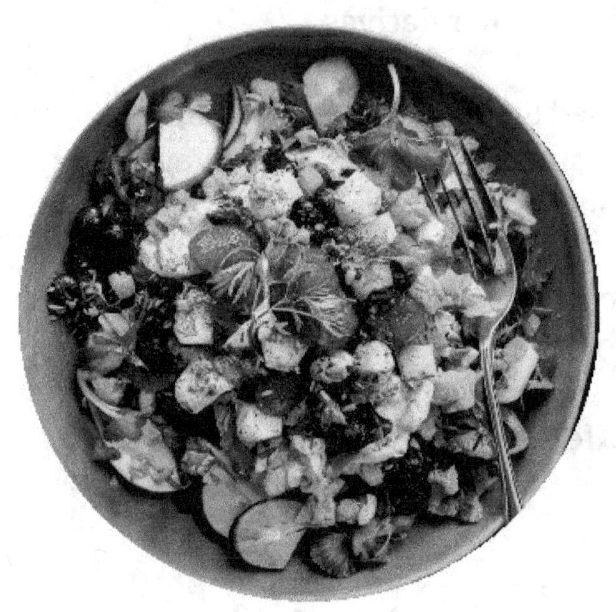

Chapter 3

The AIP Diet and Gut Health

The health of the gut is intrinsically linked to the well-being of the entire immune system. Maintaining a balanced gastrointestinal environment lies at the core of long-term autoimmune disease management through diet.

The Gut-Immune System Connection

- The gut houses over 70% of immune cells in the body in gut-associated lymphoid tissue (GALT).

- The intestinal lining acts as a semi-permeable barrier, selectively allowing nutrients to pass through while keeping pathogens out.

- When compromised by inflammation or "leaky gut", the barrier becomes overly permeable, exposing immune cells to undigested food particles.

- This erroneously signals the immune system to attack as if under foreign invasion, generating autoimmunity over time.

- The highly diverse gut microbiome interacts extensively with GALT and regulates inflammation levels systemically through metabolites produced.

How AIP Supports Gut Health

- Eliminating common food allergens gives the irritated GI tract a chance to heal without ongoing exposure/damage.

- Fermented foods plus bone broth provide probiotic bacteria and nutrients like glutamine/gelatin to repair the intestinal lining.

- Anti-inflammatory nutrition from produce, healthy fats and proteins tamps down gut inflammation at its root.

- Limiting toxins, antibiotics, NSAIDs, and stressors protects intestinal cells from further insults.

- Consumption of prebiotic fibers feeds beneficial microbes to restore diversity and balance microbial metabolism signaling in the gut and beyond.

By focusing on recovery of healthy gut function, the AIP protocol addresses a core cause of systemic inflammation behind many autoimmune illnesses. With diligent lifestyle changes, functional integrity of the gastrointestinal barrier and microbiome can return.

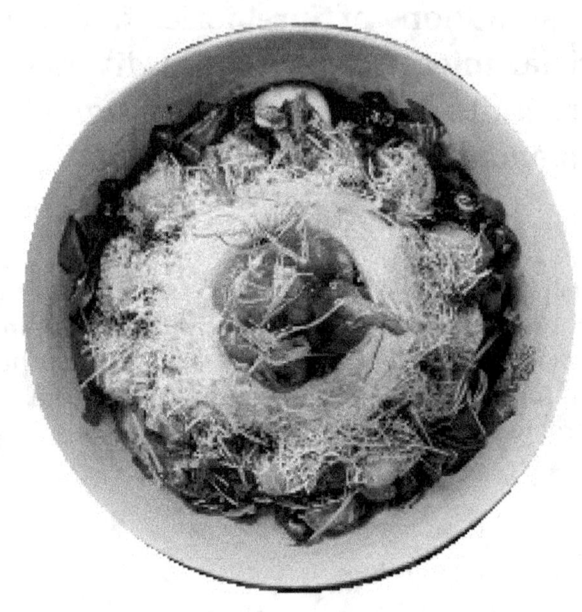

Chapter 4

The AIP Diet and Inflammation

At the crux of autoimmunity lies chronic, overactive inflammation in the body. The dietary strategies of AIP are uniquely positioned to modulate the inflammatory response through multiple avenues.

Understanding Inflammation

- Acute inflammation is a normal immune response to infection/injury that aids healing through increased blood flow and white blood cells.

- But persistent low-grade inflammation triggers autoimmune disorders by inducing collateral damage to healthy tissues over years/decades.

- Factors like genetics, smoking, stress, toxins, and food allergies can ignite and perpetuate this hyper-activated state.

How AIP Reduces Inflammation

- Eliminating top dietary triggers like gluten and dairy that promote inflammation removes a leading external cause.

- Fermented foods, prebiotics and glutamine facilitate restoring beneficial bacteria which produce short-chain fatty acids to downregulate inflammation.

- Anti-inflammatory nutrients abundant in whole foods include omega-3s, antioxidants, polyphenols, indole-3-carbinol and sulforaphane.

- Avoiding refined carbs and sugar decreases triggers for spikes and chronic elevation of inflammatory proteins through balanced blood sugar control.

- Cooking methods like boiling soup stocks emphasize anti-inflammatory compounds while minimizing Acrylamide formation during high-heat processing.

- Lifestyle factors addressed including managing stress, exposure to toxins, sleep, hydration and movement further calm the inflammatory response.

By targeting and rebalancing the root causes, AIP takes a multipronged approach proven effective at resolving the hyperinflammatory condition driving autoimmunity.

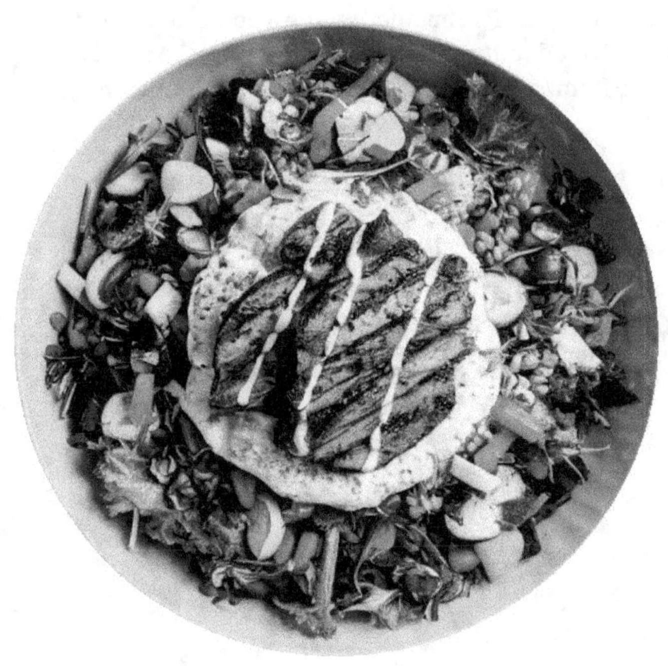

Chapter 5

The AIP Diet and Nutrient Density

Achieving optimal nutrition plays a key supporting role in autoimmune healing. The AIP framework emphasizes whole, minimally processed foods to maximize micronutrient intake.

Micronutrient Deficiencies

Certain nutrient inadequacies are common in autoimmune patients due to poor diet, malabsorption issues or drug effects on absorption. Things like:

- Vitamin D - Critical for immune regulation yet many are deficient.

- Magnesium - Important cofactor in over 300 biochemical reactions but soil depletion impacts levels.

- Vitamin B12 - Deficiency linked to inflammation, neurological damage if vegan/vegetarian.

- Omega-3s - Promote anti-inflammatory eicosanoid production but standard American diet lacks EPA/DHA.

Maximizing Nutrient Density

- Grass-fed meat/wild fish packs more nutrients than conventional and is encouraged.

- Bone broth provides collagen, glucosamine and other joint-protective molecules.

- Organ meats like liver are nutrient powerhouses but may need to be reintroduced.

- Dark leafy greens and cruciferous veggies loaded with antioxidants like vitamins C, K.

- Fermented foods enhance bioavailability through culturing, improving absorption.

- Coconut products add beneficial fats while supporting thyroid and adrenal function.

- Homemade dressings with cod or salmon oils boost heart-healthy fats.

- Healthy fats deliver fat-soluble vitamins, support cell function and satiety.

Following these principles enables autoimmune patients to obtain critical foundation from natural whole foods for repairing tissues and restoring resilience. Addressing potential deficiencies empowers the body's self-healing abilities.

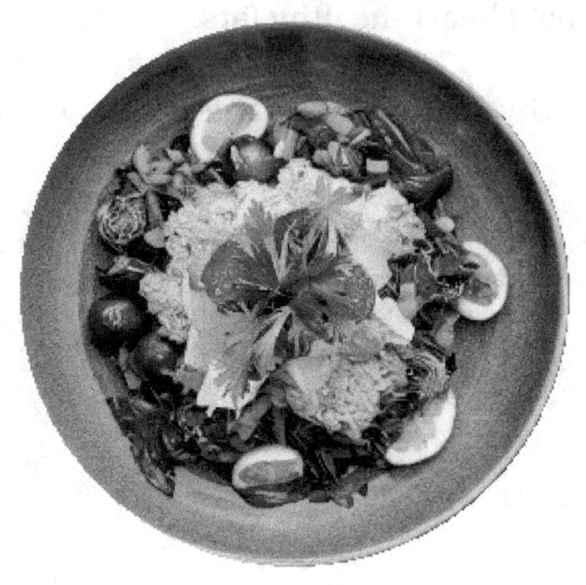

Chapter 6

Meal Planning on the AIP Diet

Thoughtful meal planning is instrumental to the long-term success and sustainability of the AIP lifestyle. Here are some helpful strategies:

Batch Cooking

- Cook extra meat, grains and veggies to repurpose for meals later in the week.

- Roast multiple chickens or prepare casseroles with leftovers in mind.

- Portion and freeze items like soups, stews and chilis for easy grab-and-go options.

Grocery List

- Plan recipes and make a detailed list to avoid impulse buys.

- Shop weekly sales and seasonal produce for variety on a budget.

- Stock up basics that don't expire like coconut products, bone broth, oils.

Meal Assembly

- Prepare breakfasts/lunches ahead of time and store them in bento boxes or containers.

- Package nuts, dried fruit, salmon oil or other snacks for on-the-go.

- Let soups simmer in a slow cooker on days when time is limited.

Mix It Up

- Rotate between easy and more involved recipes to keep enjoyment.

- Mix up protein, veggie and fat/carb sources to balance each meal.

- Plan both warm homemade meals and hearty cold salads.

Involve Others

- Meal prep can feel like a chore solo - delegate tasks or cook together for family support.

- Involve kids by letting them help prepare age-appropriate parts of recipes.

Consistent meal planning sets you up for dietary success with zero excuses. Staying fueled with nutritious, compliant dishes prevents backsliding or overwhelming cravings.

---

30 Days Meal Planner

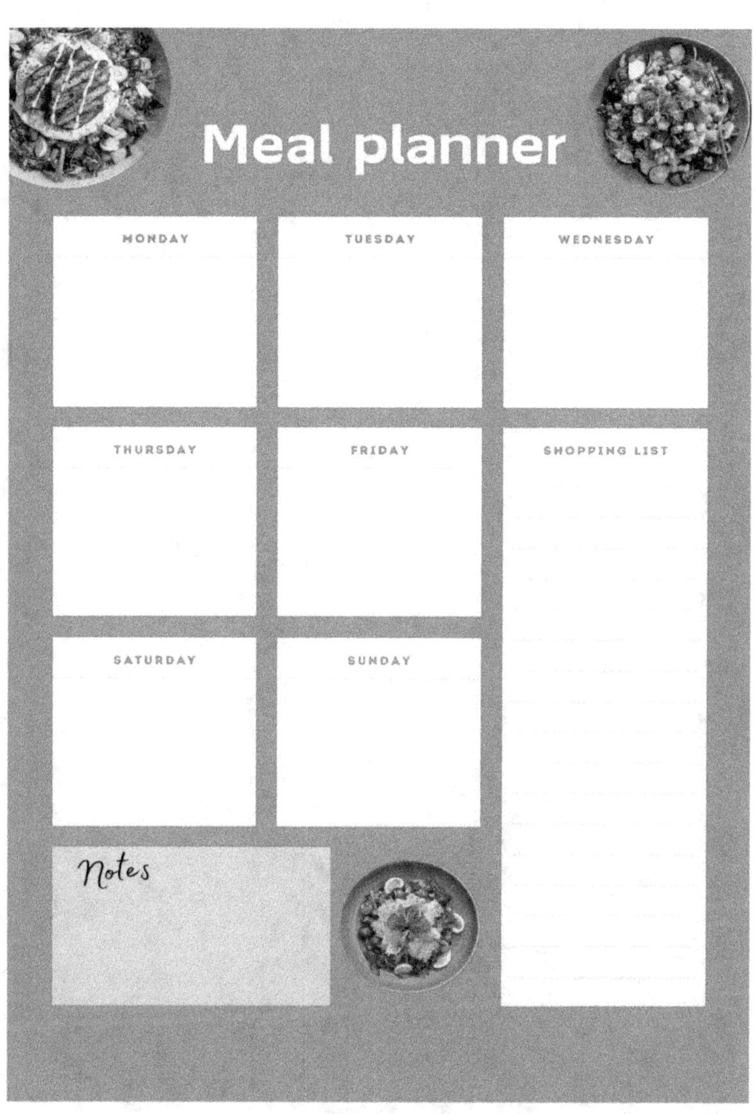

Meal planner
MONDAY
TUESDAY
WEDNESDAY
THURSDAY
FRIDAY
SHOPPING LIST
SATURDAY
SUNDAY
Notes

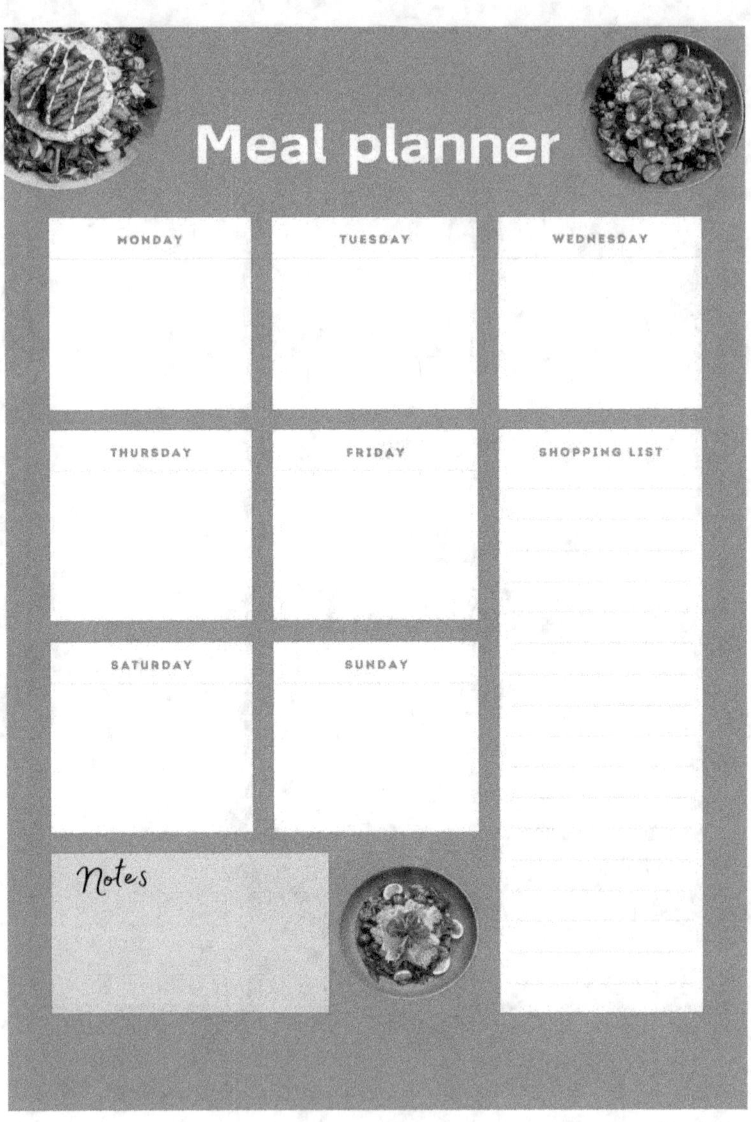

Meal planner
MONDAY
TUESDAY
WEDNESDAY
THURSDAY
FRIDAY
SHOPPING LIST
SATURDAY
SUNDAY
Notes

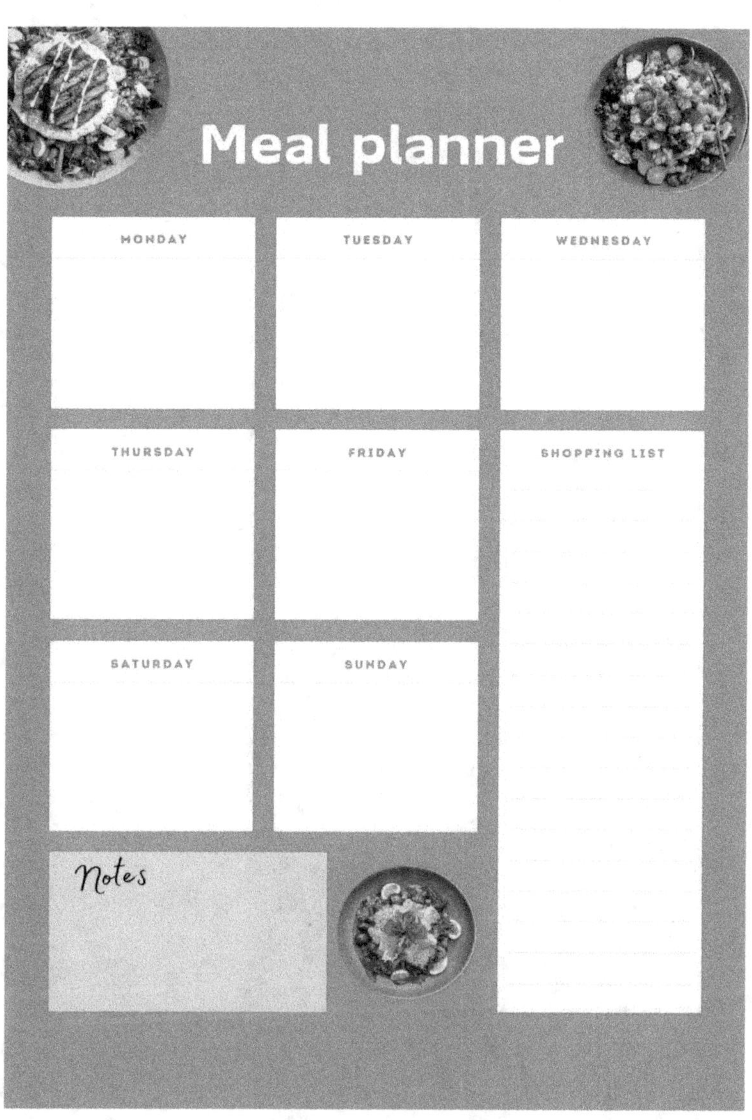
Meal planner
MONDAY
TUESDAY
WEDNESDAY
THURSDAY
FRIDAY
SHOPPING LIST
SATURDAY
SUNDAY
Notes

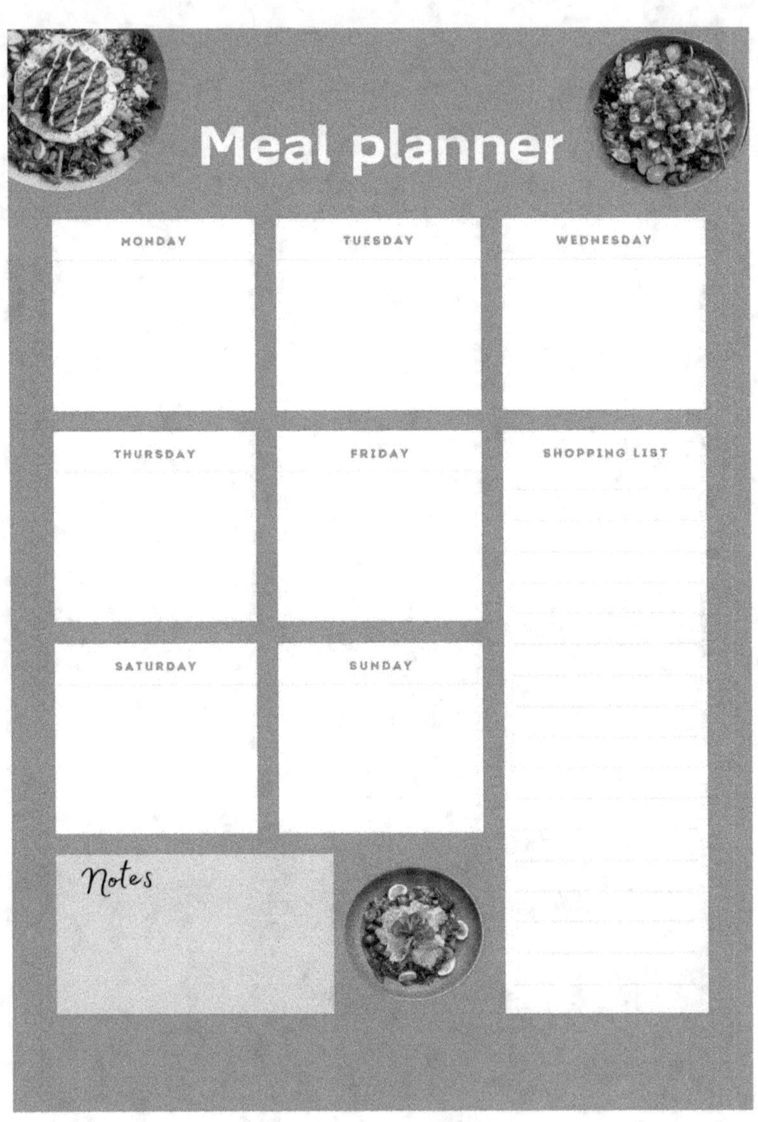
Meal planner
MONDAY
TUESDAY
WEDNESDAY
THURSDAY
FRIDAY
SHOPPING LIST
SATURDAY
SUNDAY
Notes

Meal planner

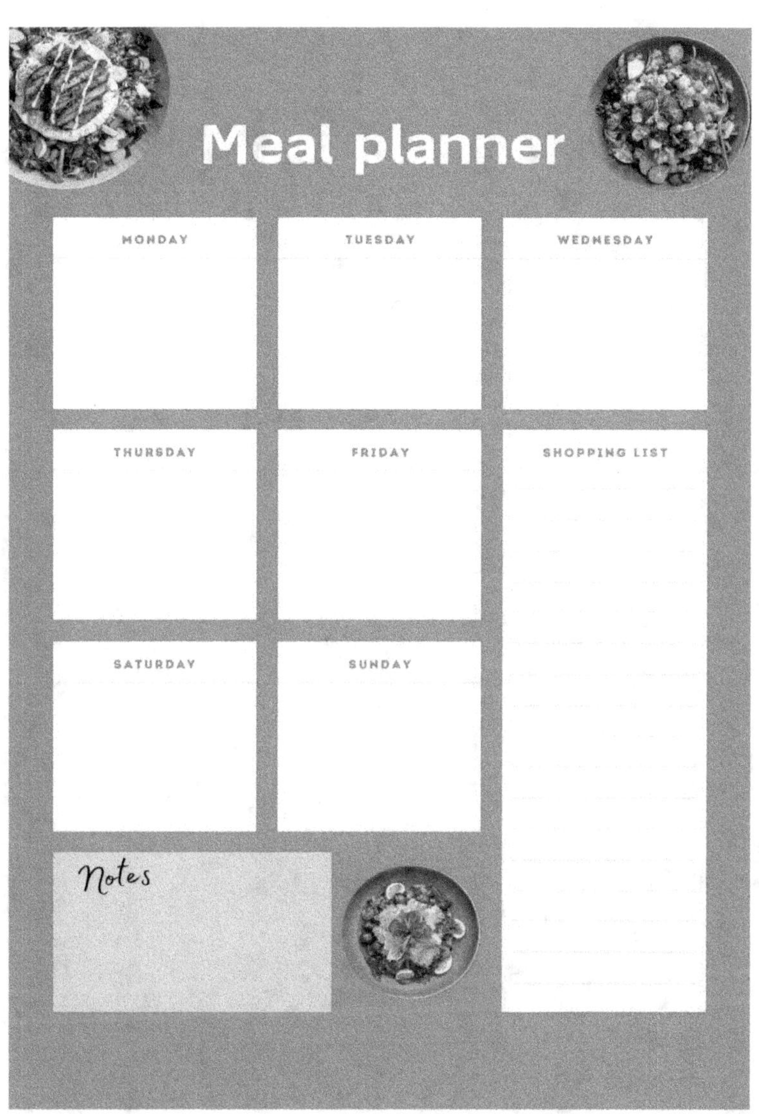

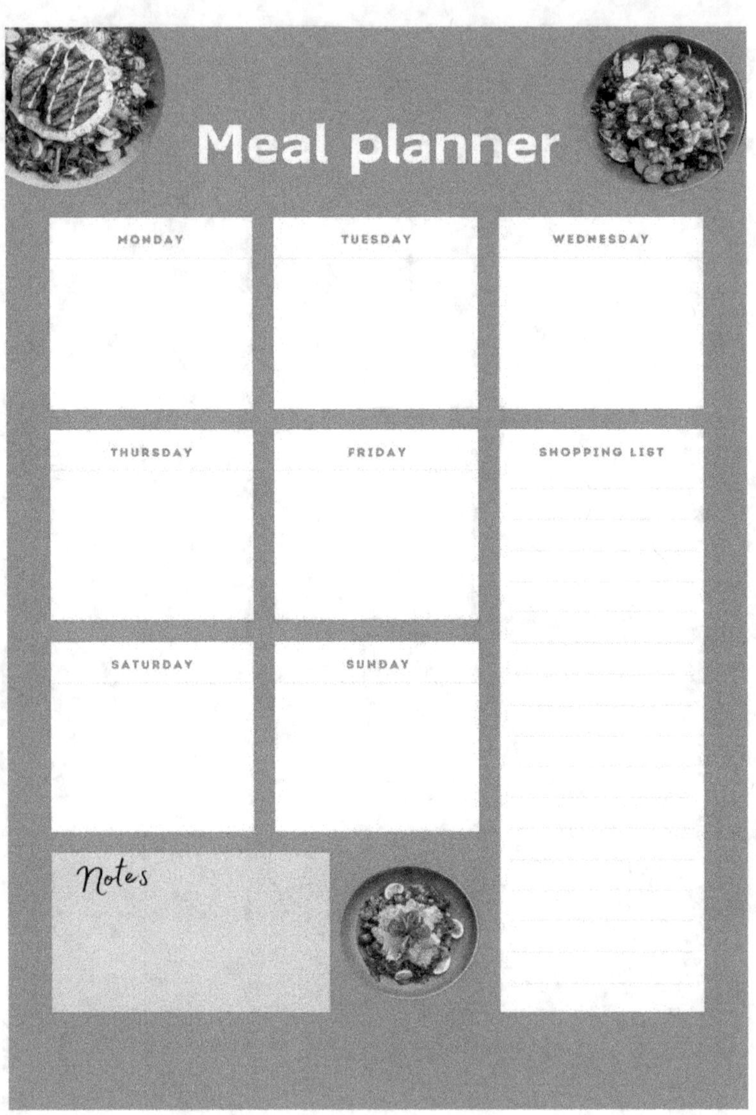

Meal planner
MONDAY
TUESDAY
WEDNESDAY
THURSDAY
FRIDAY
SHOPPING LIST
SATURDAY
SUNDAY
Notes

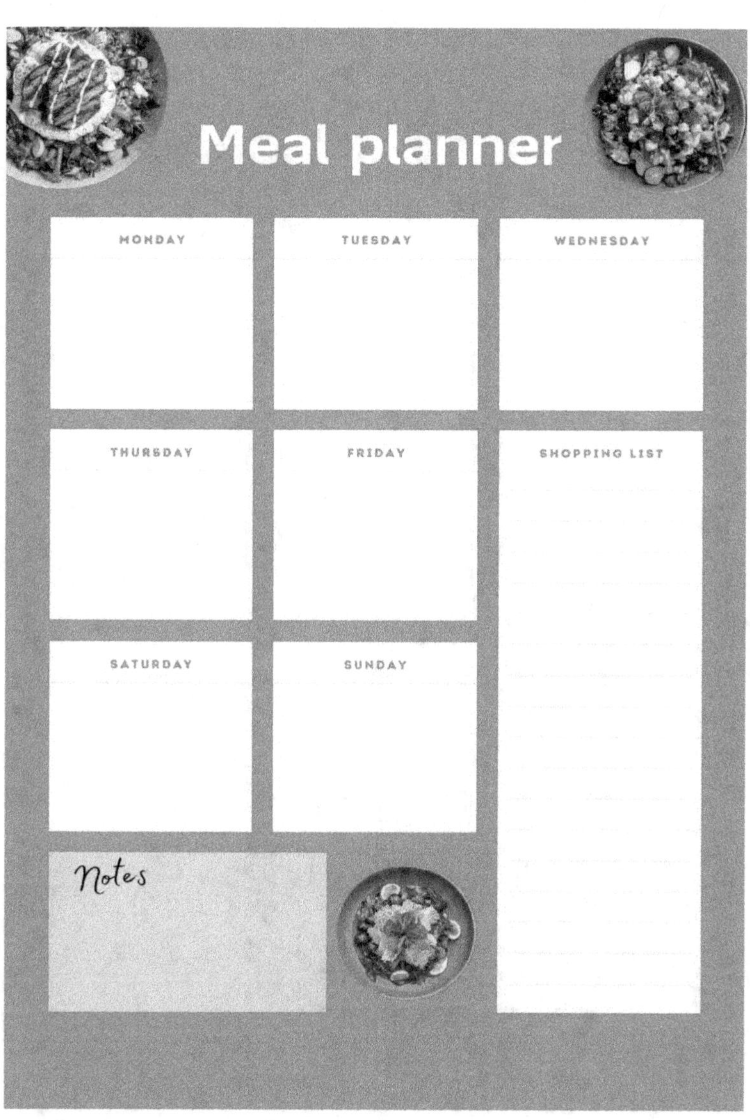

Meal planner
MONDAY
TUESDAY
WEDNESDAY
THURSDAY
FRIDAY
SHOPPING LIST
SATURDAY
SUNDAY
Notes

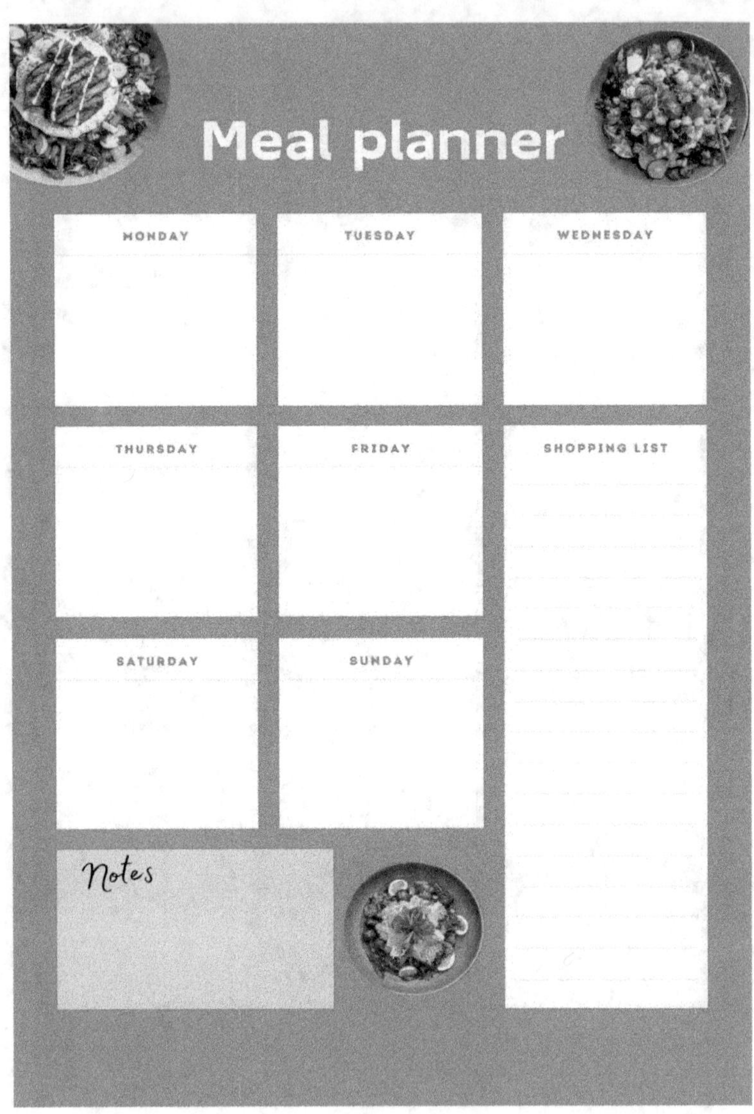
Meal planner
MONDAY
TUESDAY
WEDNESDAY
THURSDAY
FRIDAY
SHOPPING LIST
SATURDAY
SUNDAY
Notes

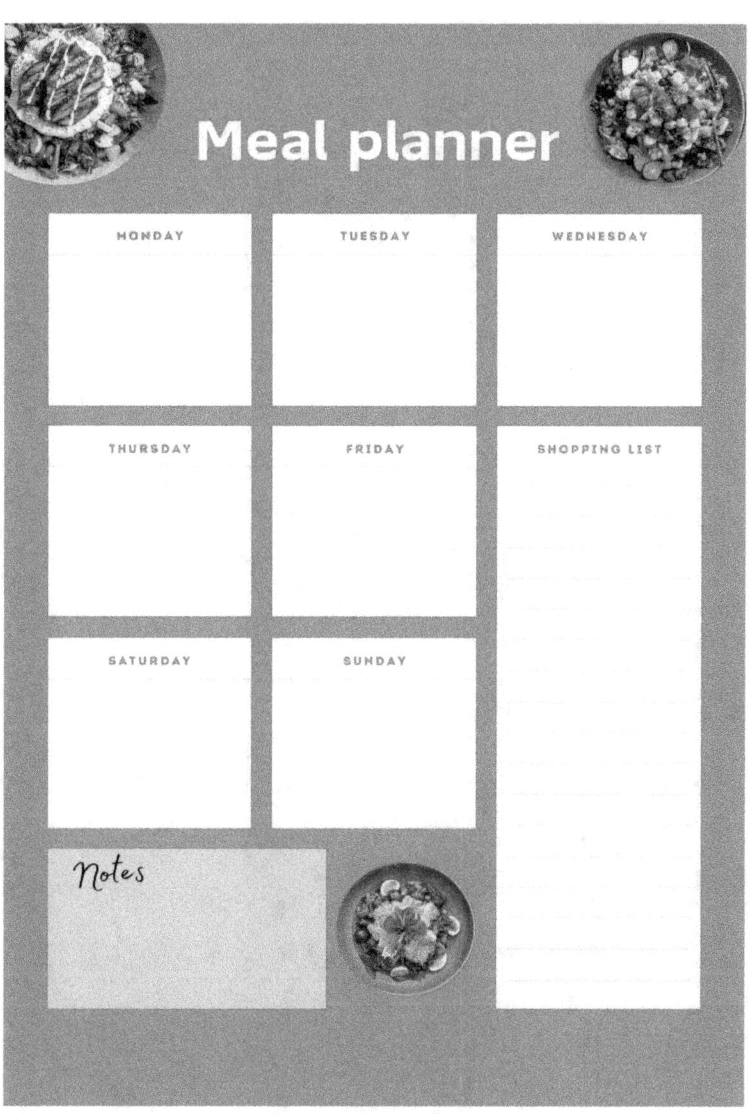

Meal planner
MONDAY
TUESDAY
WEDNESDAY
THURSDAY
FRIDAY
SHOPPING LIST
SATURDAY
SUNDAY
Notes

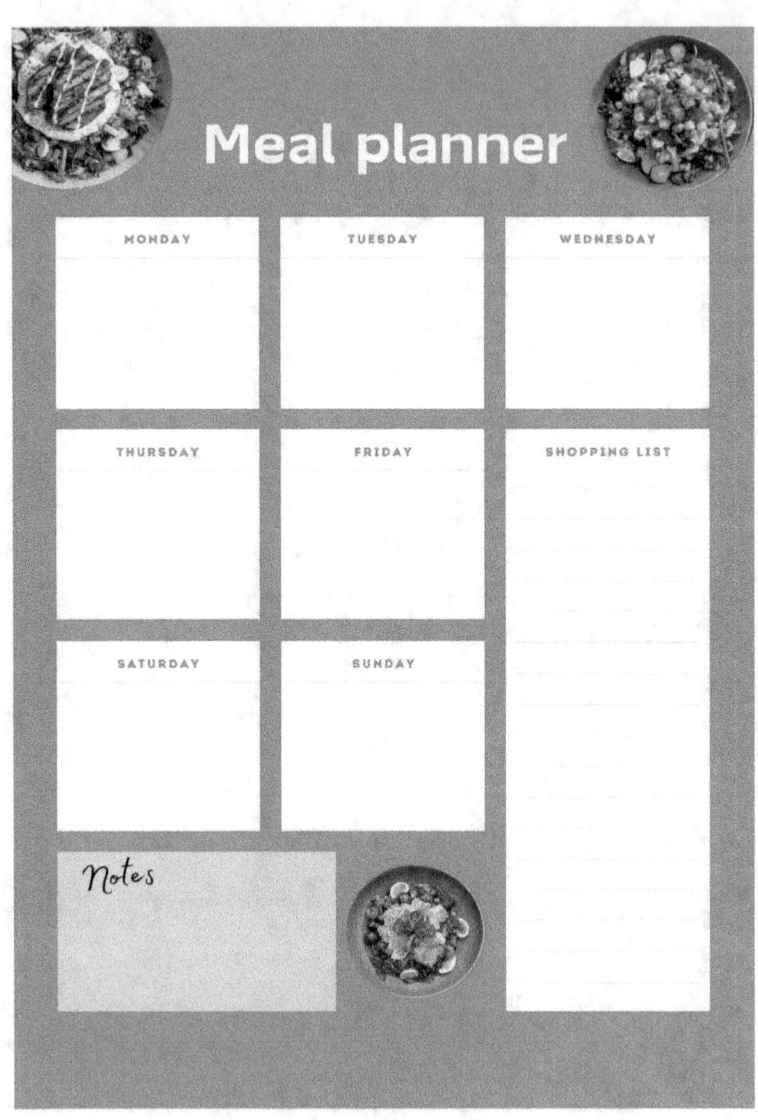

Meal planner
MONDAY
TUESDAY
WEDNESDAY
THURSDAY
FRIDAY
SHOPPING LIST
SATURDAY
SUNDAY
Notes

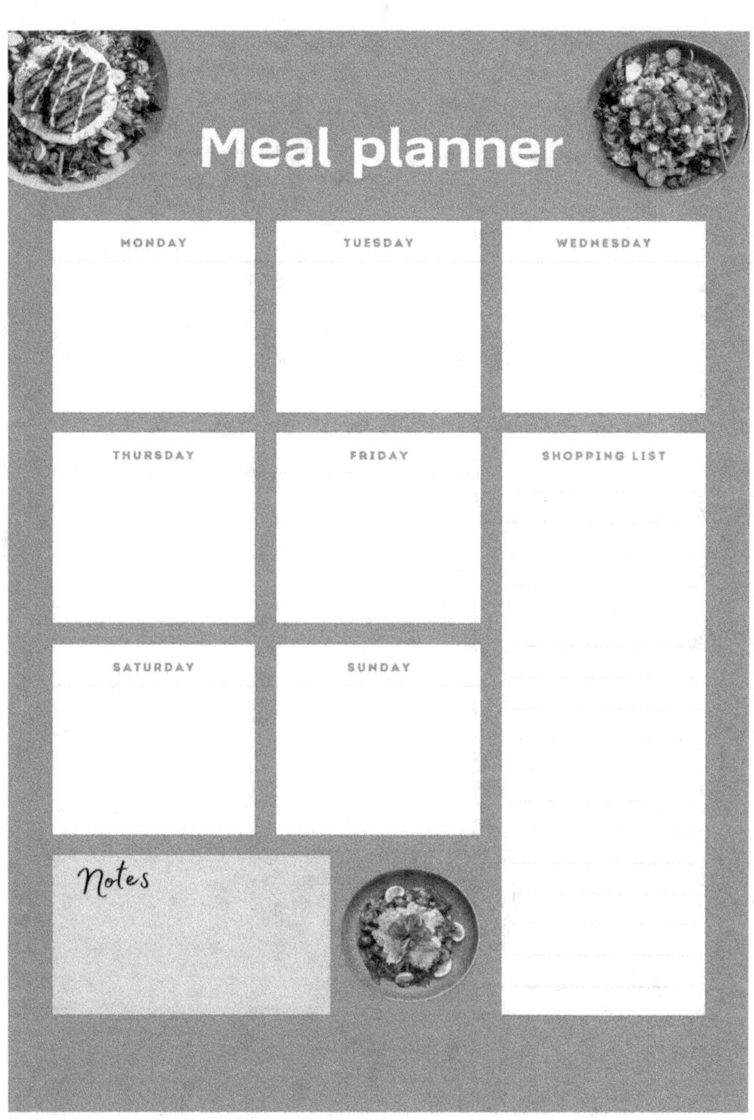

Meal planner
MONDAY
TUESDAY
WEDNESDAY
THURSDAY
FRIDAY
SHOPPING LIST
SATURDAY
SUNDAY
Notes

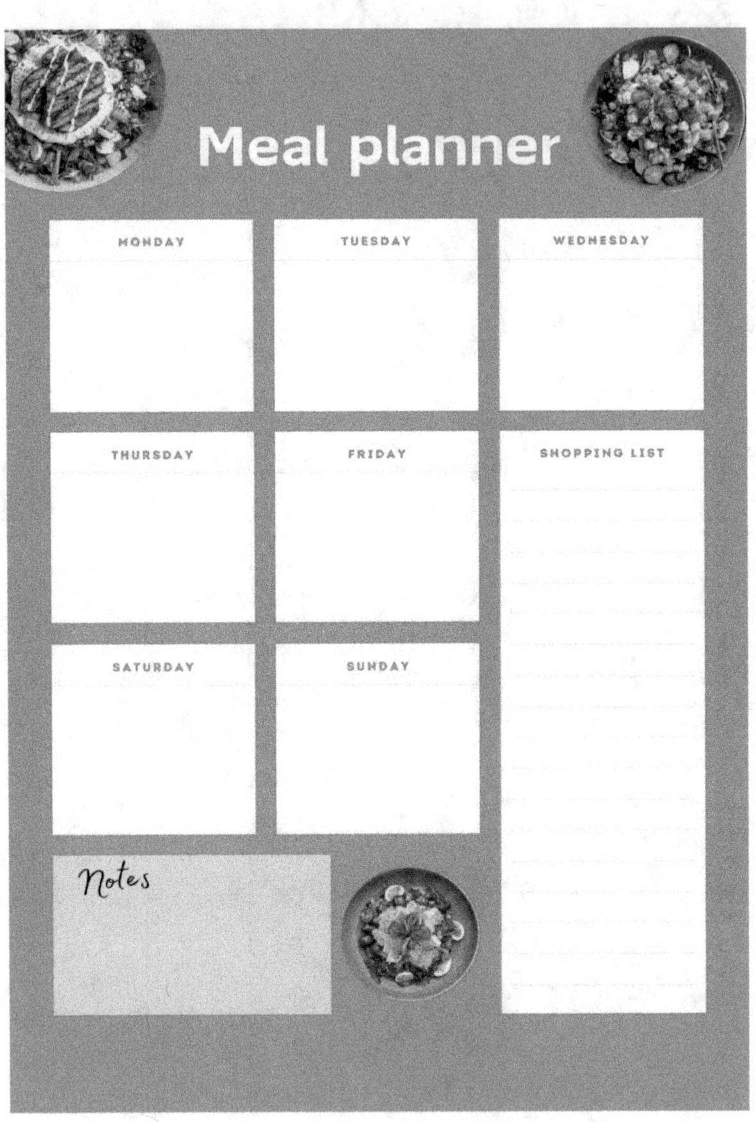
Meal planner
MONDAY
TUESDAY
WEDNESDAY
THURSDAY
FRIDAY
SHOPPING LIST
SATURDAY
SUNDAY
Notes

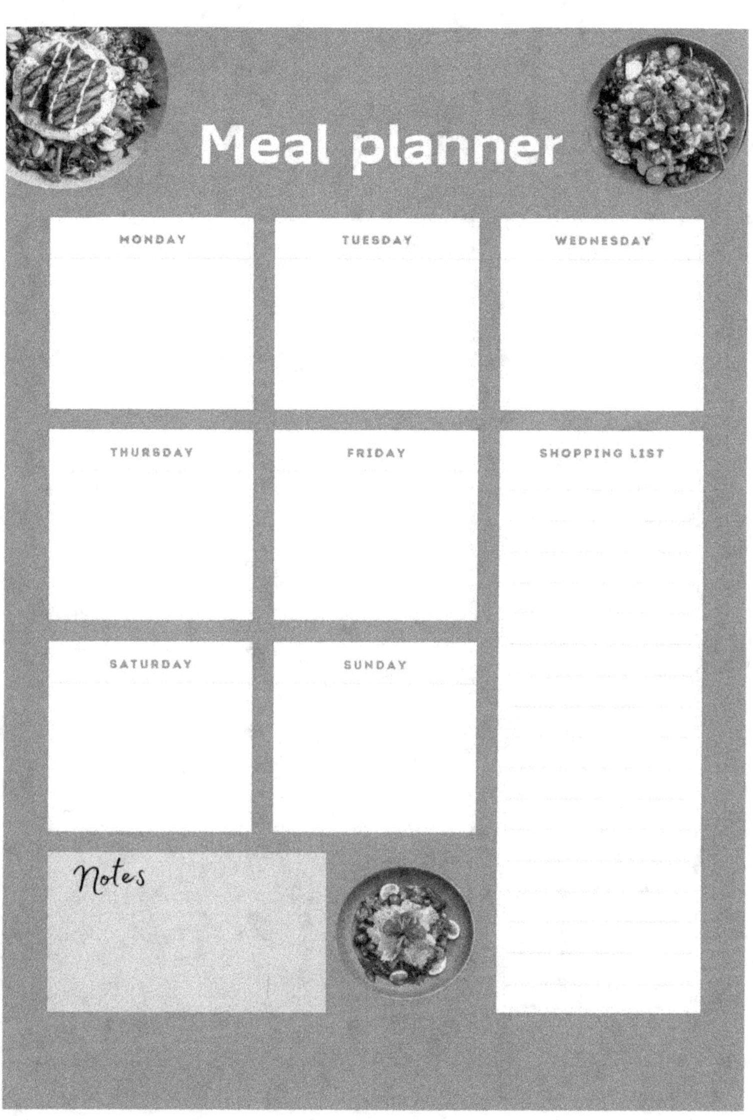

Meal planner
MONDAY
TUESDAY
WEDNESDAY
THURSDAY
FRIDAY
SHOPPING LIST
SATURDAY
SUNDAY
Notes

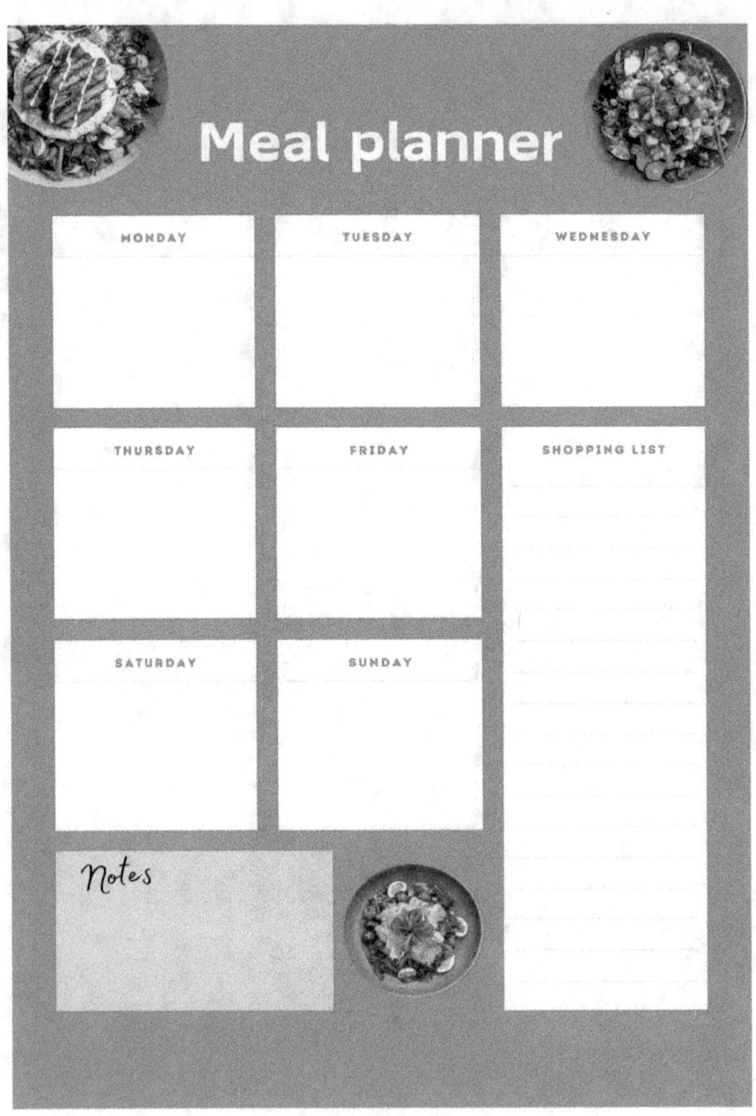

Meal planner
MONDAY
TUESDAY
WEDNESDAY
THURSDAY
FRIDAY
SHOPPING LIST
SATURDAY
SUNDAY
Notes

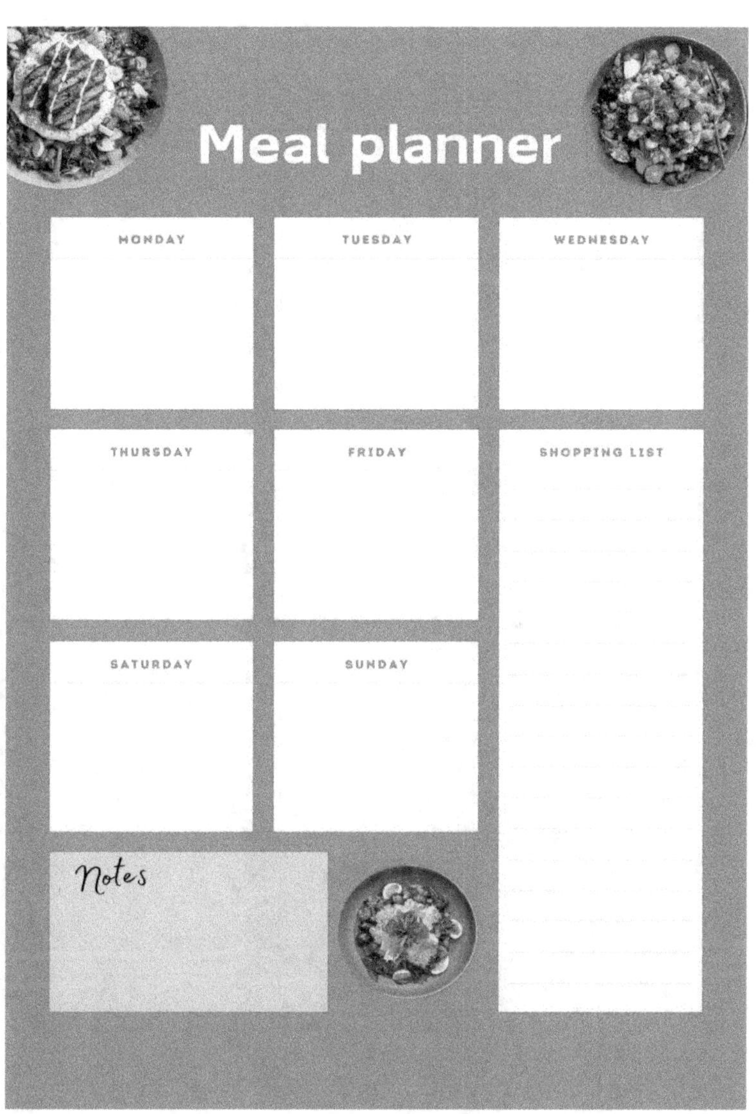

Meal planner
MONDAY
TUESDAY
WEDNESDAY
THURSDAY
FRIDAY
SHOPPING LIST
SATURDAY
SUNDAY
Notes

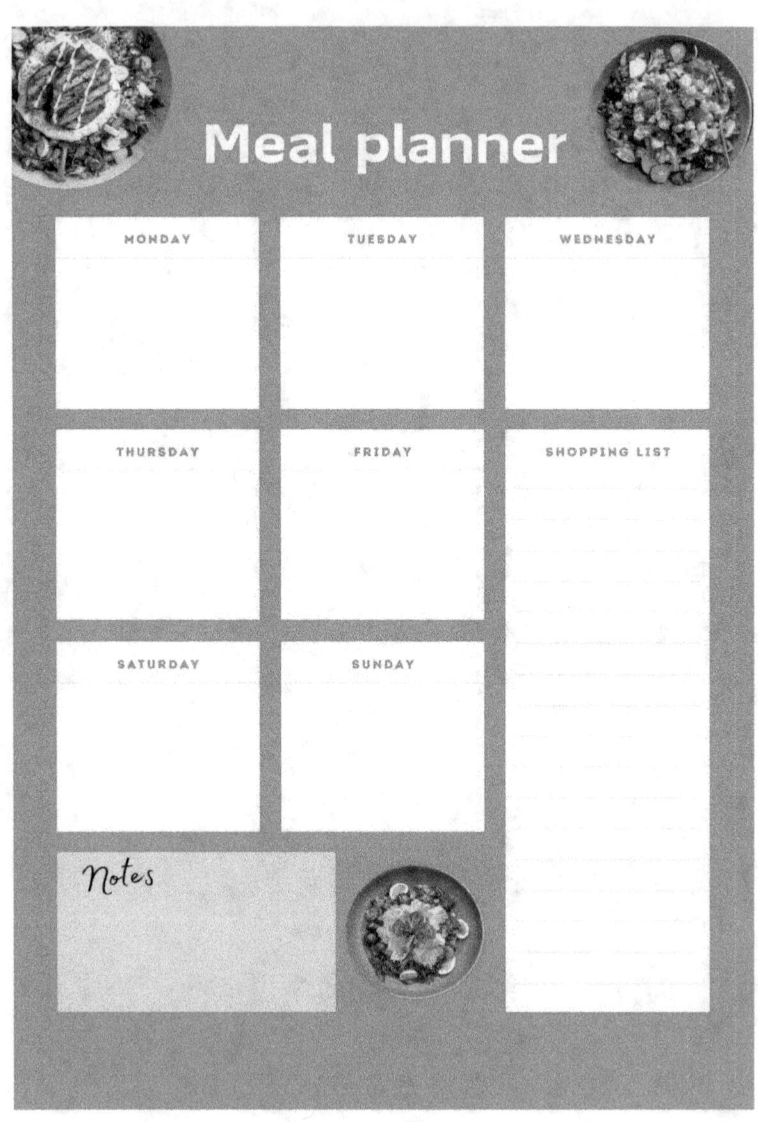

Meal planner
MONDAY
TUESDAY
WEDNESDAY
THURSDAY
FRIDAY
SHOPPING LIST
SATURDAY
SUNDAY
Notes

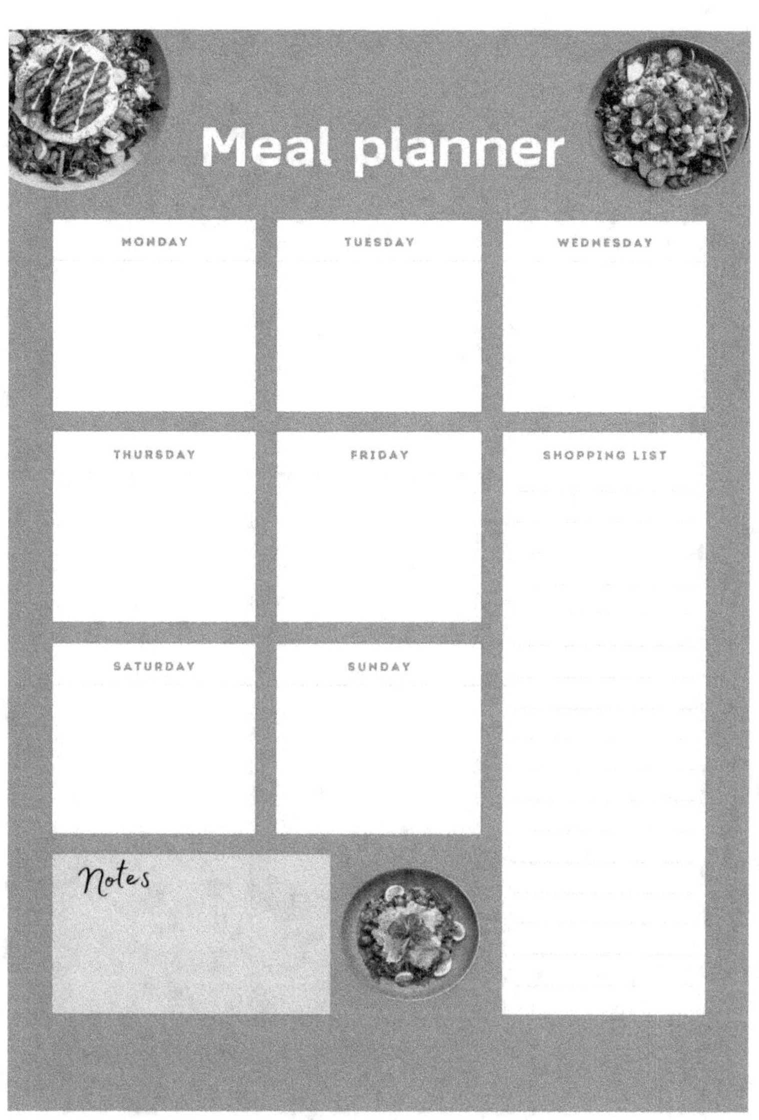

Meal planner
MONDAY
TUESDAY
WEDNESDAY
THURSDAY
FRIDAY
SHOPPING LIST
SATURDAY
SUNDAY
Notes

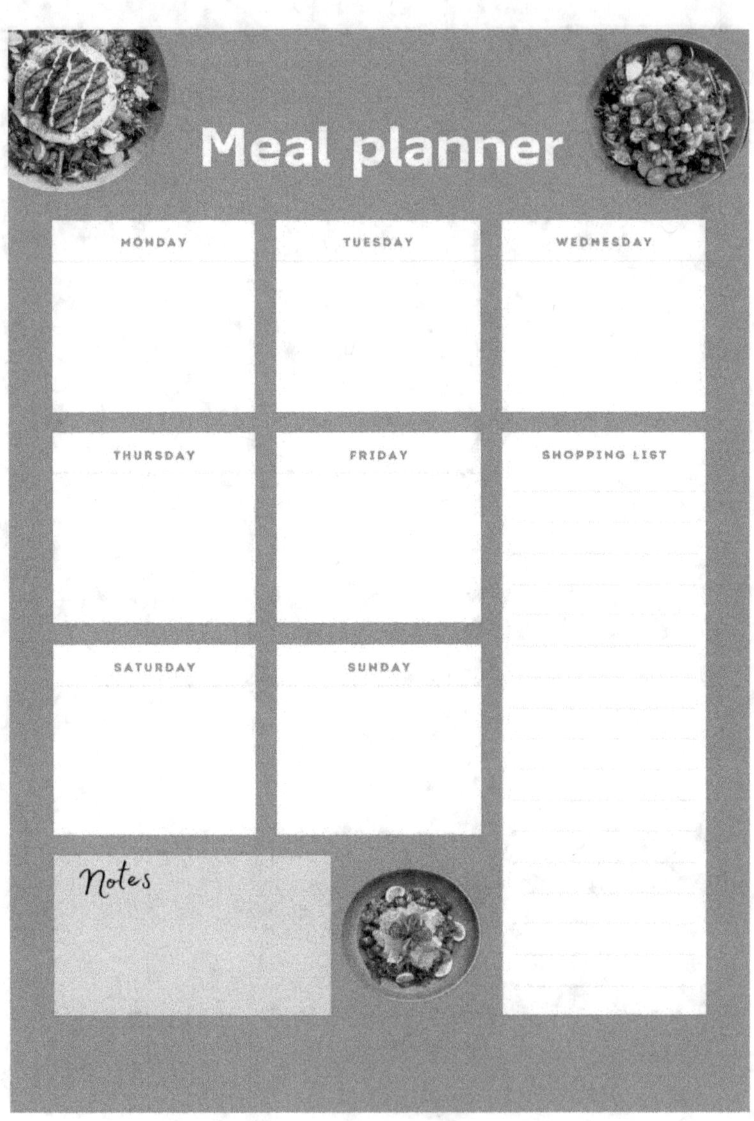

Meal planner
MONDAY
TUESDAY
WEDNESDAY
THURSDAY
FRIDAY
SHOPPING LIST
SATURDAY
SUNDAY
Notes

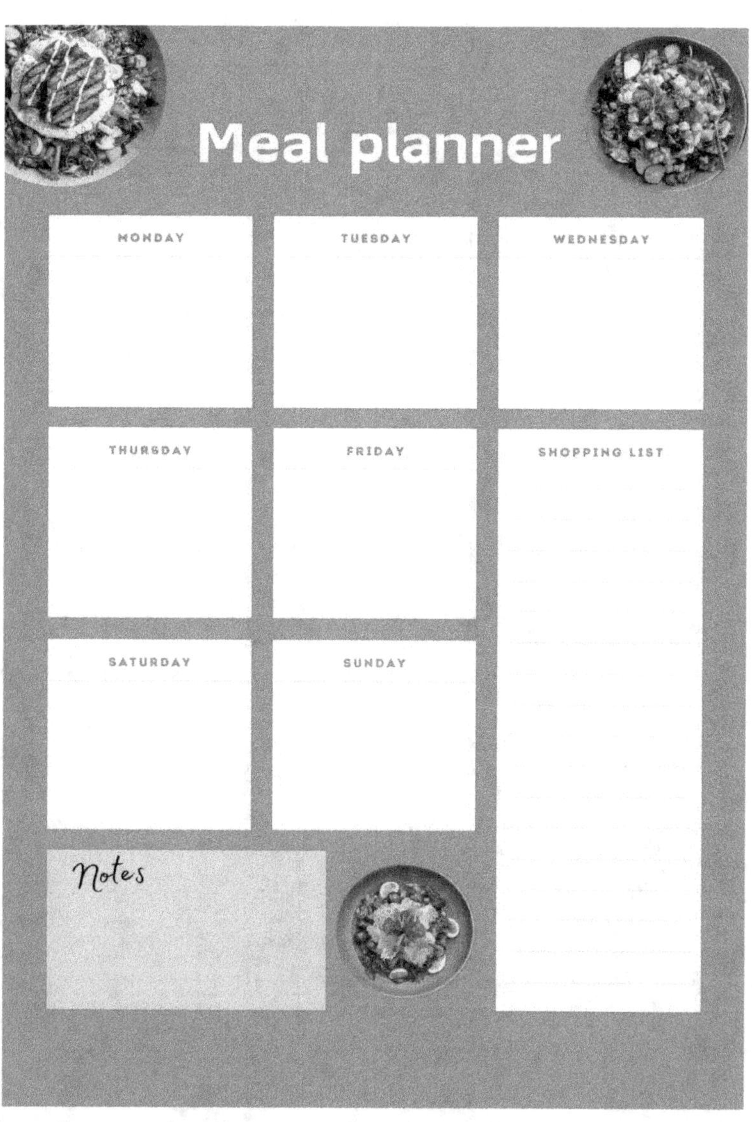

Meal planner
MONDAY
TUESDAY
WEDNESDAY
THURSDAY
FRIDAY
SHOPPING LIST
SATURDAY
SUNDAY
Notes

Meal planner

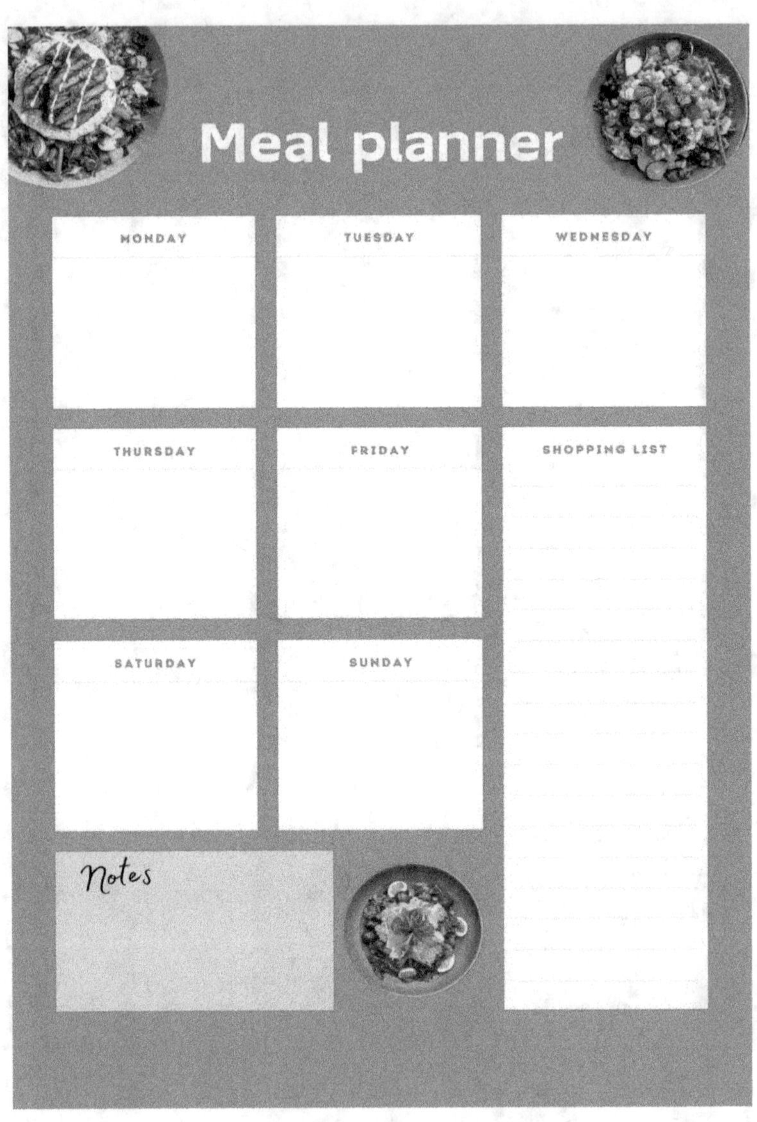

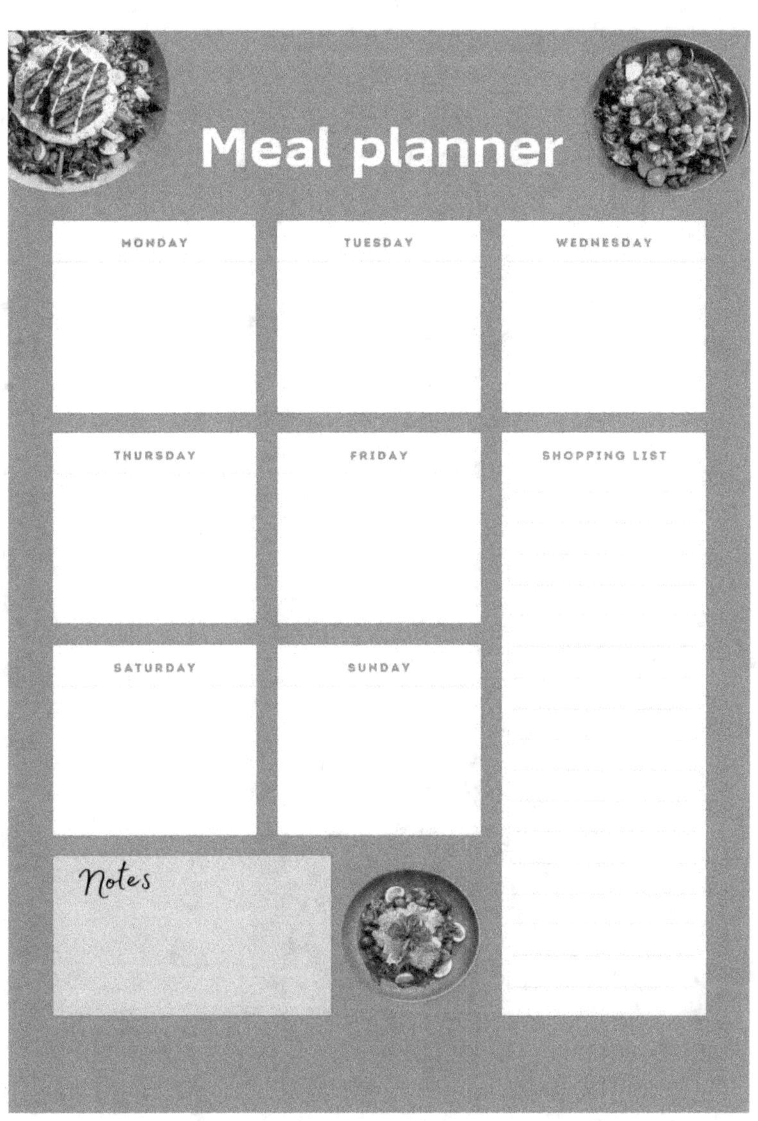

Meal planner
MONDAY
TUESDAY
WEDNESDAY
THURSDAY
FRIDAY
SHOPPING LIST
SATURDAY
SUNDAY
Notes

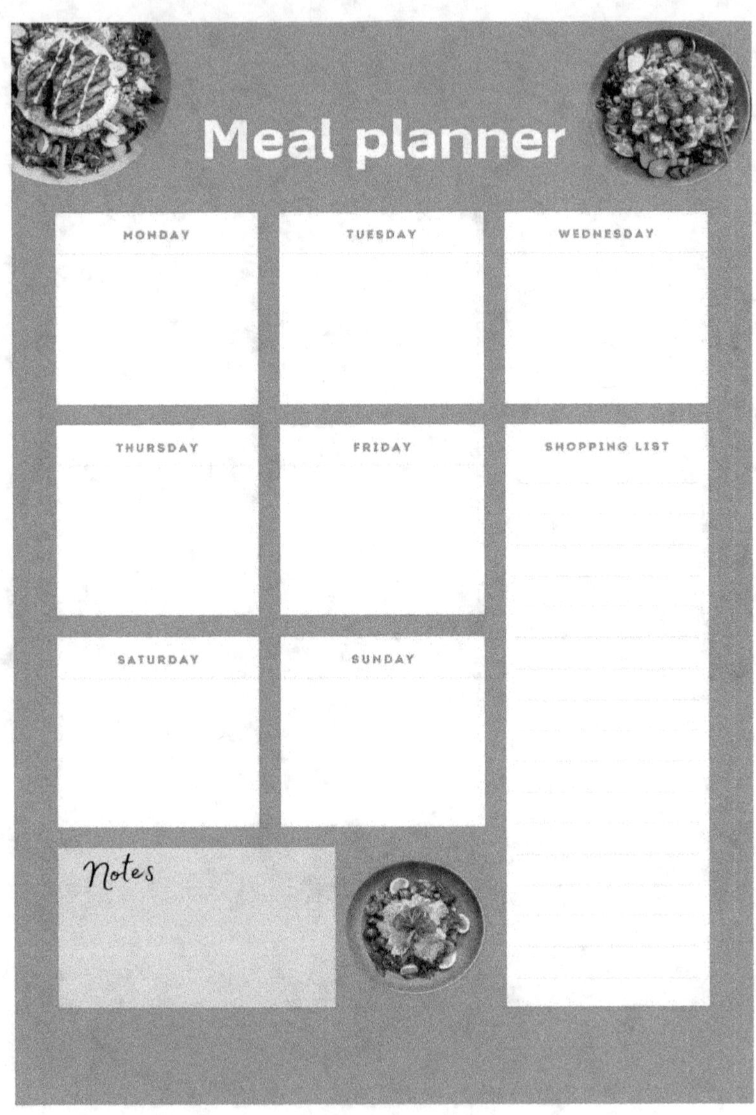
Meal planner
MONDAY
TUESDAY
WEDNESDAY
THURSDAY
FRIDAY
SHOPPING LIST
SATURDAY
SUNDAY
Notes

Meal planner

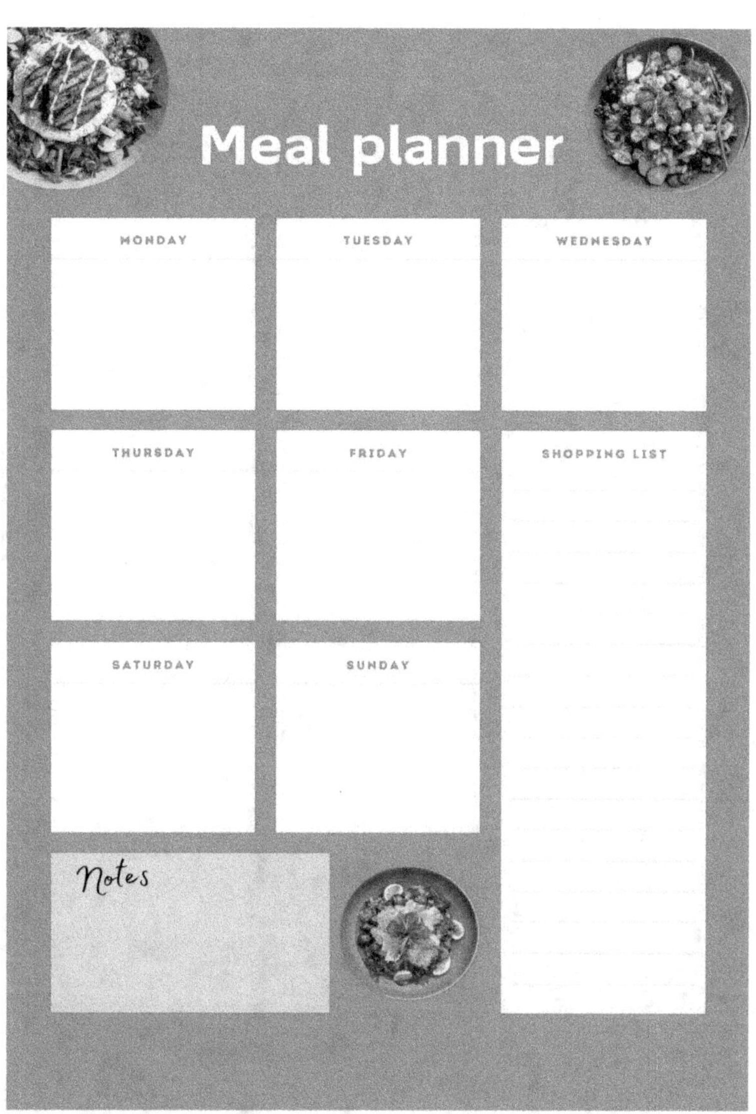

Meal planner

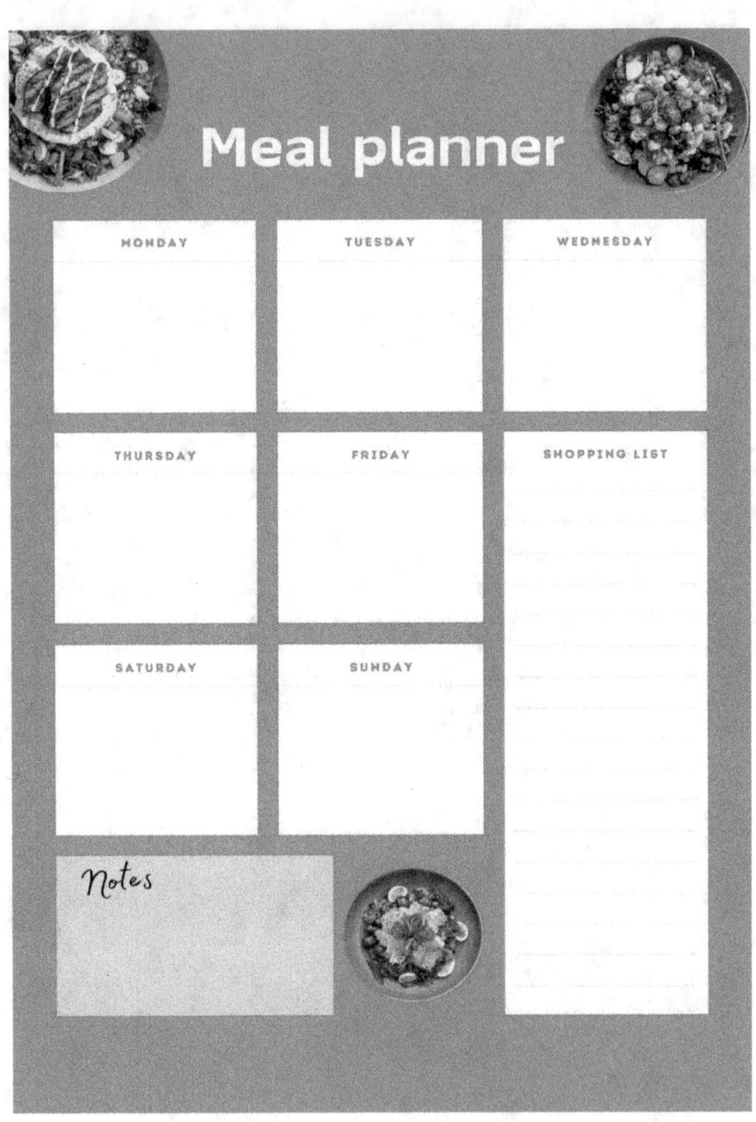

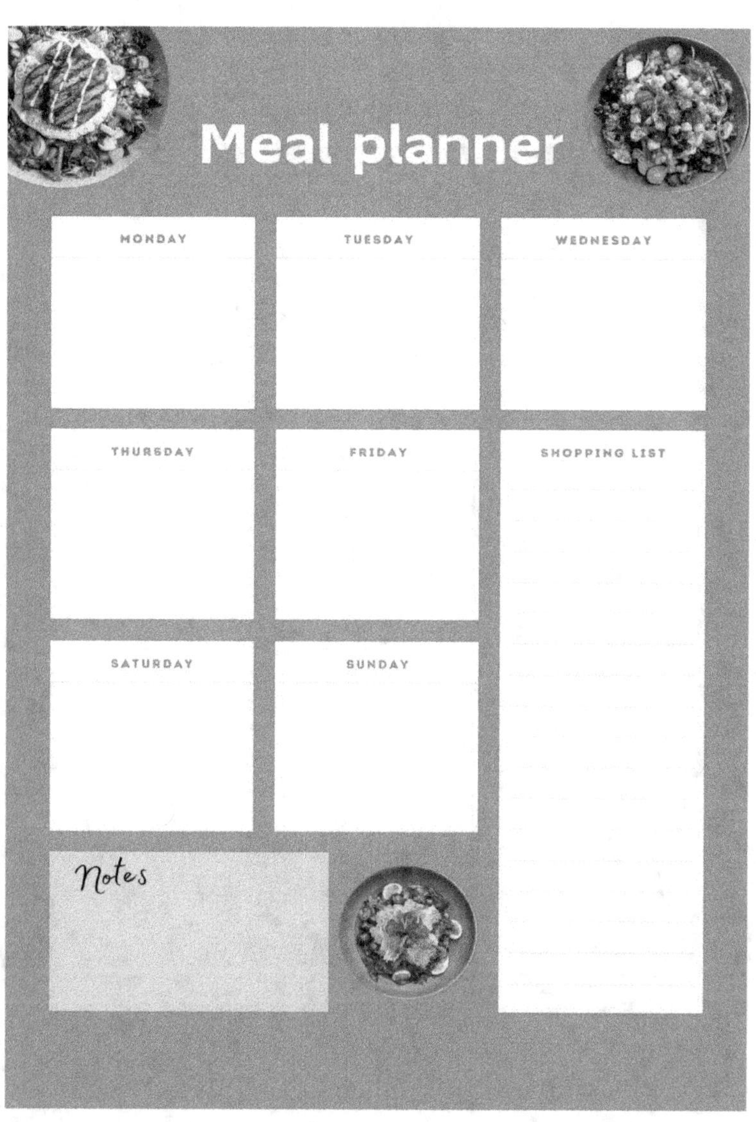

Meal planner
MONDAY
TUESDAY
WEDNESDAY
THURSDAY
FRIDAY
SHOPPING LIST
SATURDAY
SUNDAY
Notes

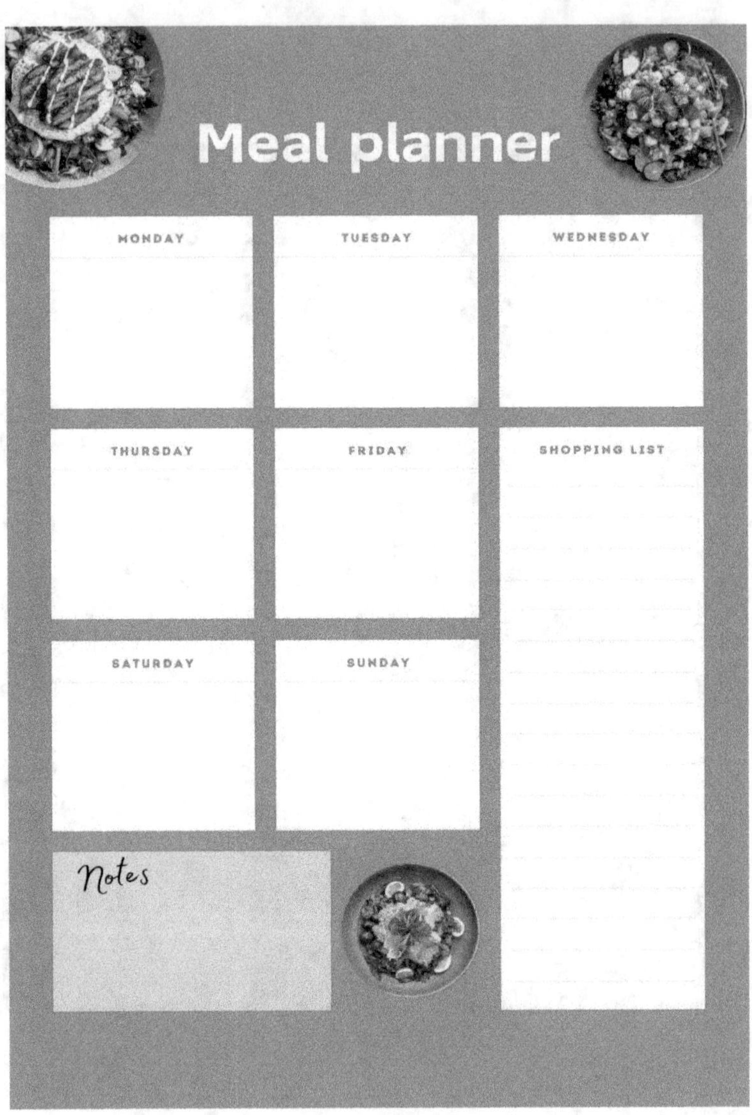

Meal planner
MONDAY
TUESDAY
WEDNESDAY
THURSDAY
FRIDAY
SHOPPING LIST
SATURDAY
SUNDAY
Notes

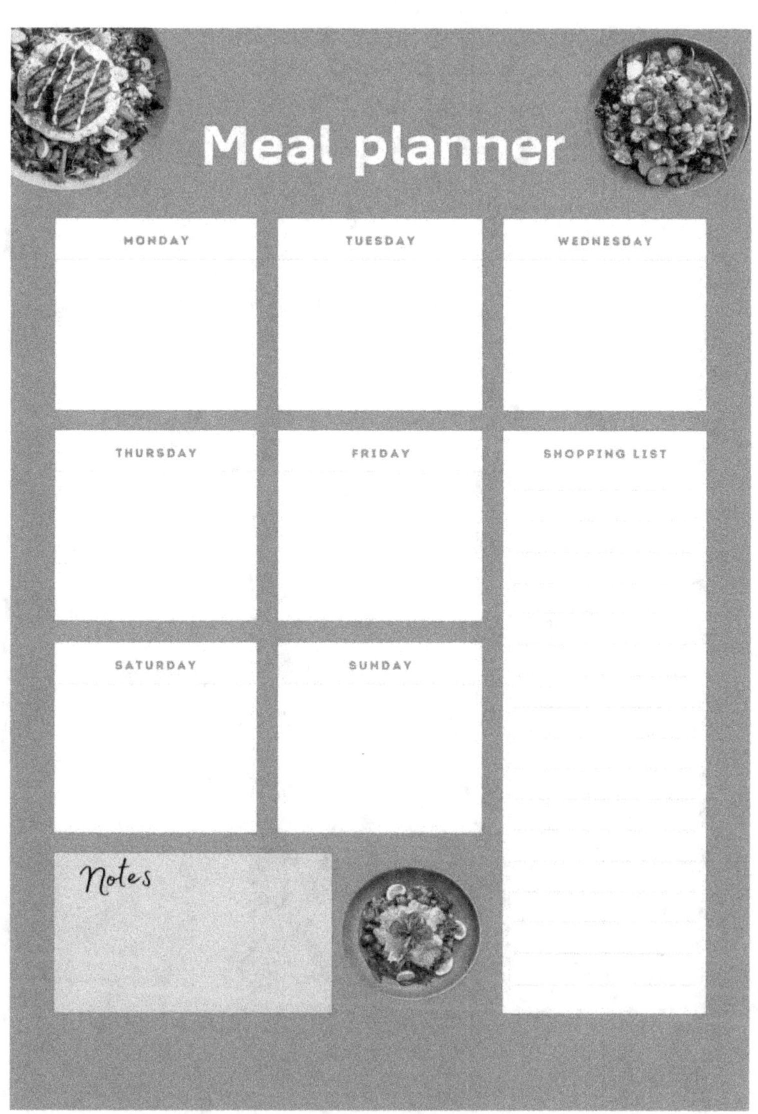

Meal planner
MONDAY
TUESDAY
WEDNESDAY
THURSDAY
FRIDAY
SHOPPING LIST
SATURDAY
SUNDAY
Notes

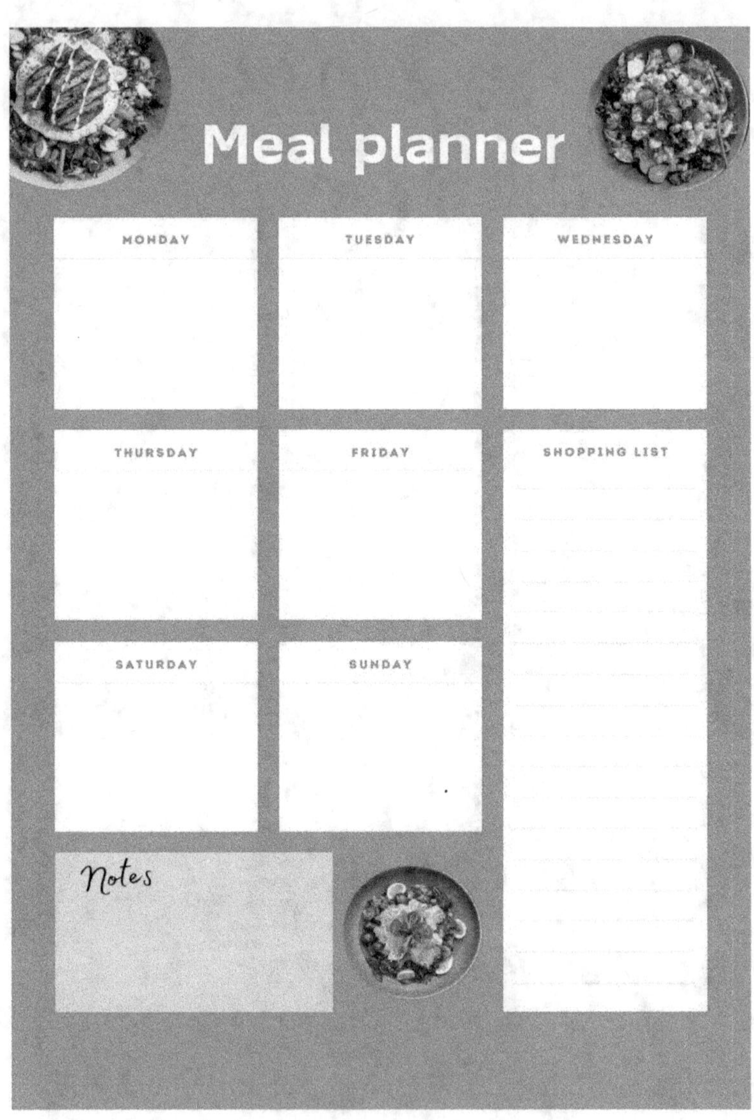

Meal planner
MONDAY
TUESDAY
WEDNESDAY
THURSDAY
FRIDAY
SHOPPING LIST
SATURDAY
SUNDAY
Notes

Meal planner

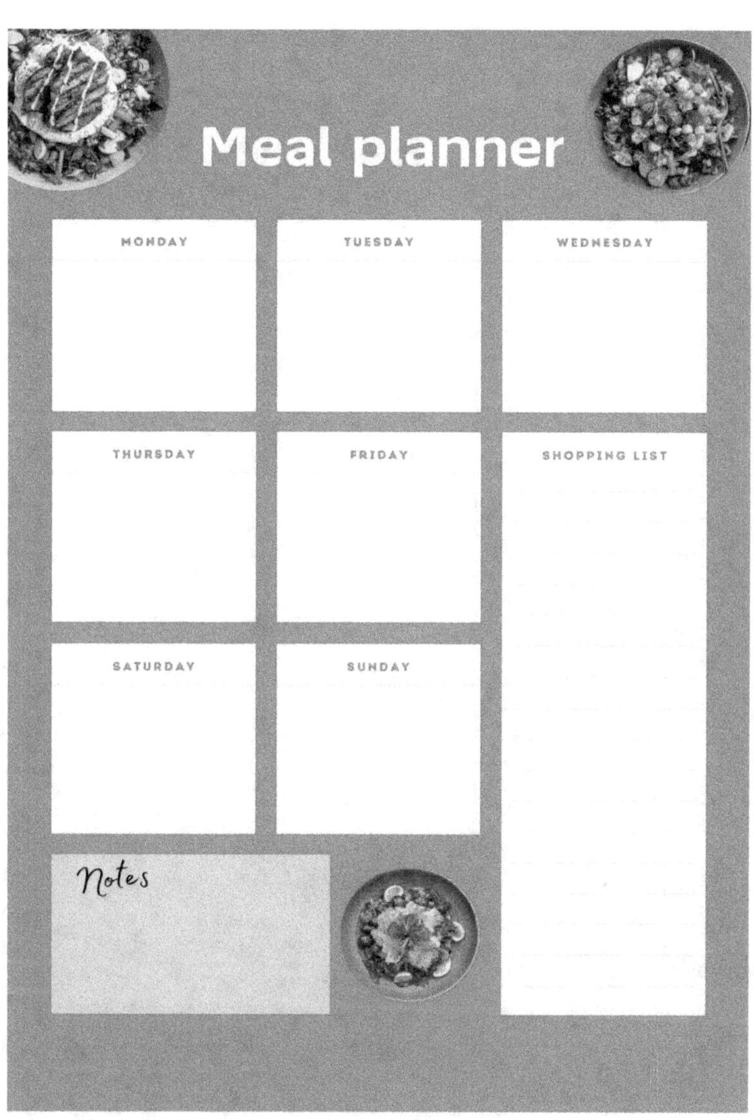

Meal planner

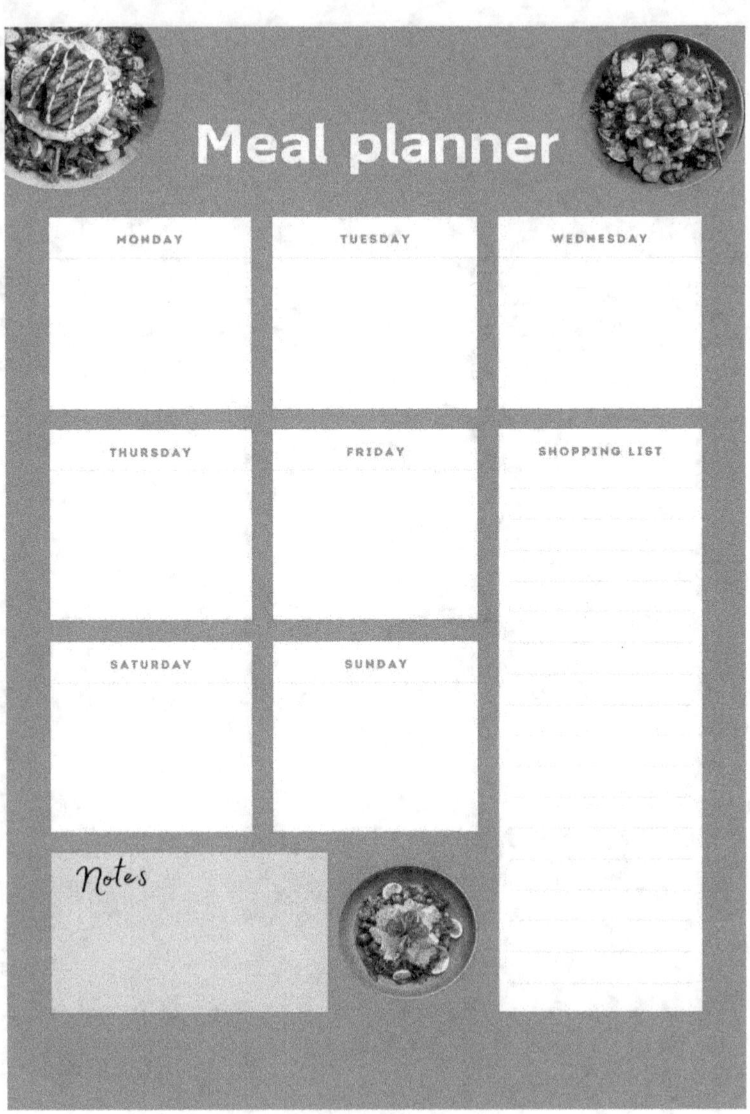

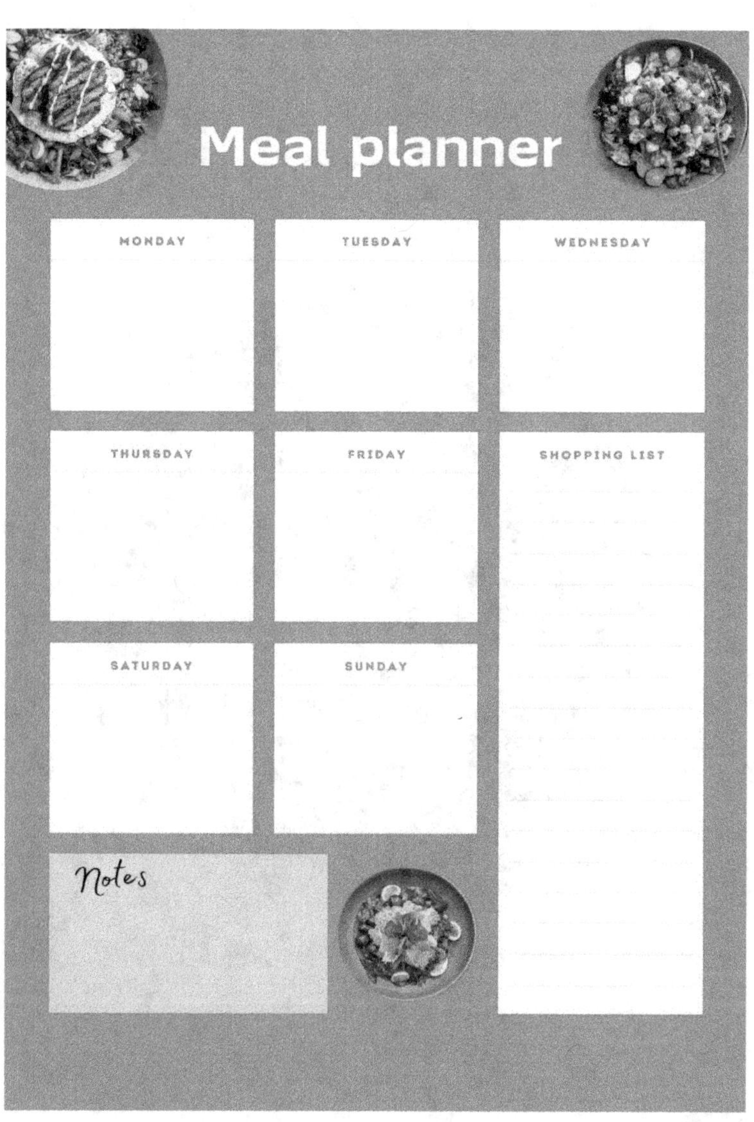

Meal planner

MONDAY
TUESDAY
WEDNESDAY
THURSDAY
FRIDAY
SHOPPING LIST
SATURDAY
SUNDAY
Notes

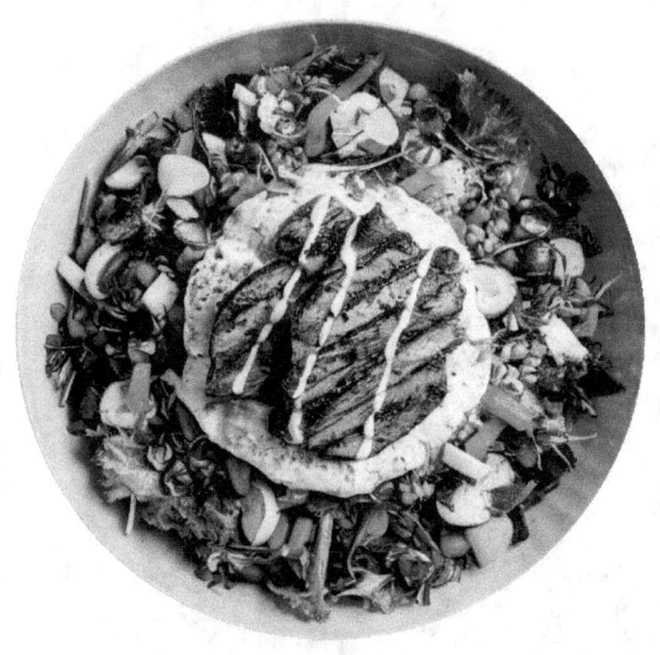

Chapter 7

Cooking Techniques for the AIP Diet

How food is prepared impacts nutrient density as well as potential inflammation. Low and slow cooking aligns well with AIP principles.

Sautéing and Stir-Frying

- Uses small amounts of heart-healthy fat over medium-high heat to quickly cook ingredients.

- Coconut, avocado and ghee are good choices. Go lightly to avoid overcooking nutrients.

Steaming

- A simple technique using a steamer basket to cook foods in the vapor from simmering water below.

- Highly effective for vegetables to retain most nutrients and flavors with little clean-up.

Braising and Stew Cooking

- Long, slow simmering of meats and vegetables submerged in aromatic broth or wine.

- Transforms tough cuts tender while infusing nutrients from bones into broth.

Roasting and Baking

- Cooking in the dry heat of the oven caramelizes natural sugars and develops flavor complexity.

- Good for root veggies, squash, meats, etc. Watch closely to avoid burning.

Pressure Cooking
- Uses trapped steam heat to cook quicker than conventional methods while sealing in moisture.

- Soups, grains and tough vegetables are transformed in a fraction of the time deliciously.

Additionally, emphasize anti-inflammatory methods like fermenting, bone broth simmering and avoid charring, deep frying or use of refined oils. Cooking smart amplifies the healing benefits of each nutrient-dense whole food.

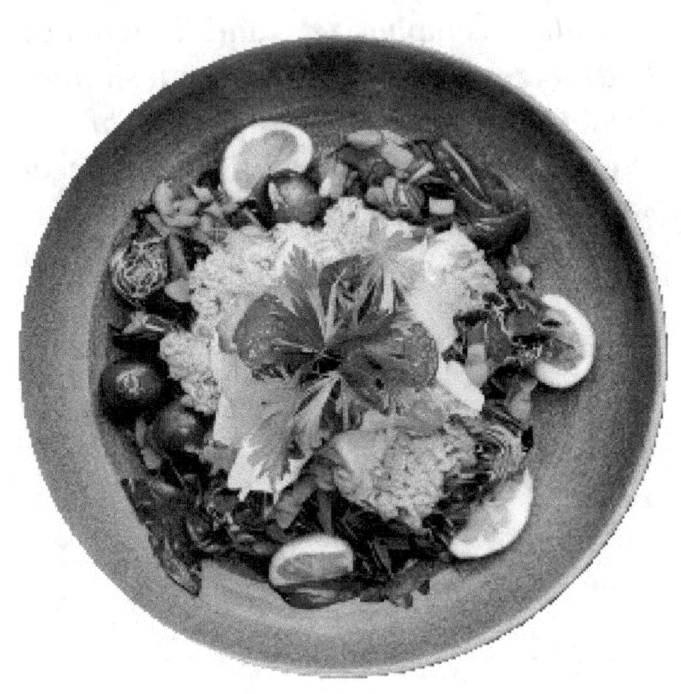

Chapter 7

Here are some delicious and nutritious AIP breakfast recipes with detailed instructions:

AIP Coconut Yogurt

Ingredients: 1 can full-fat coconut milk, 1 probiotic capsule

Method:

1. Refrigerate coconut milk overnight so it separates into solid and liquid parts.

2. Scoop out thick coconut cream and place in a bowl. Discard remaining liquid.

3. Crack open a probiotic capsule and mix the contents into coconut cream.

4. Beat with a hand mixer until smooth and creamy, about 5 minutes.

5. Transfer to an airtight container. Refrigerate 2+ hours before eating.

Nutrition: 100 calories, 11g fat, 0.5g carbs, 1g protein per 1/4 cup

<u>*Baked Eggs in Avocado*</u>

Ingredients: 1 avocado per person, 2 eggs per person

Method:

1. Preheat the oven to 375°F. Cut avocados in half and remove pits.

2. Crack 1-2 eggs into each avocado cavity. Season as desired.

3. Place on a baking sheet and bake for 20 minutes, until the egg is set.

Nutrition: 260 calories, 22g fat, 6g carbs, 11g protein per serving

Breakfast Casserole

Ingredients: 2 sweet potatoes, 1 lb kale or spinach, 8 eggs, 1 lb breakfast sausage
Method:
1. Cook and crumble sausage. Steam sweet potato and kale until soft.
2. Grease a 9x13 casserole dish. Layer ingredients and pour eggs over top.
3.Bake at 350°F for 30-40 minutes until eggs are set.
Nutrition: 495 calories, 28g fat, 30g carbs, 24g protein per serving

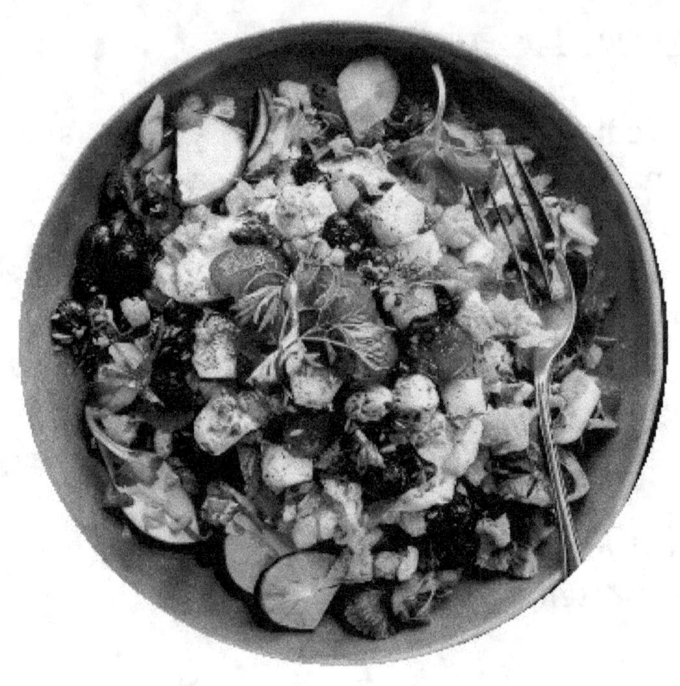

Chapter 8

Here are some delicious AIP main dish and side recipes with full instructions and nutrition:

Slow Cooker Pulled Pork

Ingredients: 2 lb pork shoulder, 1 cup bone broth, 1 onion
Method:
1. Season pork with salt and pepper. Place in a slow cooker. Top with onion slices and broth.
2. Cook on low for 8 hours. Shred with forks. Serves 6.
Nutrition (per serving): 170 calories, 6g fat, 2g carbs, 23g protein

Chicken Stir Fry

Ingredients: 1 lb chicken, 1 zucchini, 1 carrot, 1/2 bell pepper

Method:

1. Slice veggies. Cook chicken, tossing, in coconut oil for 5 minutes. Remove from the pan.

2. Stir fry veggies for 5 minutes. Return chicken to the pan and stir for 2 more minutes.

Nutrition (per serving): 200 calories, 7g fat, 6g carbs, 27g protein

Roasted Brussels Sprouts

Ingredients: 1 lb Brussels sprouts, 2 tbsp olive oil, salt and pepper
Method:
1. Toss Brussels sprouts with olive oil and seasonings.
2. Spread on a baking sheet and roast at 400°F for 25-30 minutes.
Nutrition (per serving): 80 calories, 5g fat, 6g carbs, 3g protein

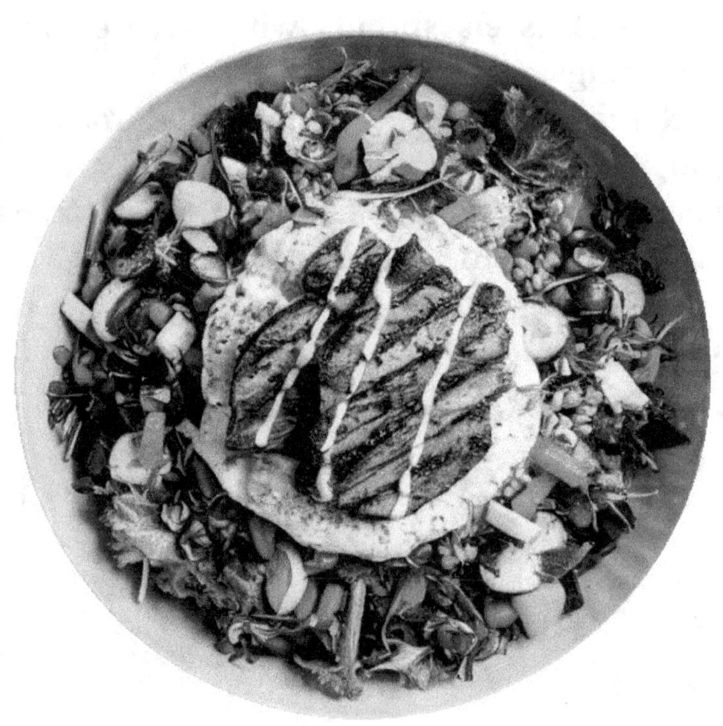

Chapter 9

Here are some delicious AIP snack and dessert recipes:

Chicken Liver Pate

- Blend chicken livers, olive oil, herbs and lemon juice until smooth. Spread on cucumber slices.

Fruit and Nut Trail Mix

- Combine 1/2 cup each of raisins, cranberries, walnuts and pumpkin seeds. Sweetened with dried coconut shreds.

Herb-Infused Chia Seed Pudding

- Whisk 1/4 cup chia seeds with 1 cup nut milk. Stir in 1 tbsp honey and 1/2 tsp vanilla. Top with berries.

Roasted Roots

- Toss beets, carrots and sweet potato with oil and roast at 400°F until tender. Season with salt and dill.

Coconut Macaroons

- Process 1 cup shredded coconut with 1/2 cup almond butter, 1/4 cup honey and 1 egg white. Drop by spoonful onto a baking sheet. Bake at 325°F for 15 minutes.

Chocolate Avocado Mousse

- Blend 1 ripe avocado, 1/4 cup cocoa, 1/3 cup honey or maple syrup, 1 tsp vanilla and pinch salt until smooth. Top with coconut shreds.

Blueberry Almond Bites

- Mix 1 cup almond flour, 1/4 cup maple syrup and 1/3 cup butter. Form into balls, press with toothpick, dip in chopped blueberries. Bake at 350°F for 10 minutes.

AIP DIET RECIPES

Here's a more comprehensive outline for the "Guide to Quick, Easy, and Delicious Low-Carb Recipes for a Healthy and Vibrant Life." We'll start with several categories and provide a few recipes under each category. The categories could include appetizers, main dishes, sides, and desserts.

Guide to Quick, Easy, and Delicious Low-Carb Recipes for a Healthy and Vibrant Life

Table of Contents

1. Appetizers
   - Garlic Butter Shrimp
   - Caprese Salad
   - Avocado Deviled Eggs
2. Main Dishes
   - Baked Lemon Herb Salmon
   - Chicken Alfredo Spaghetti Squash
   - Zucchini Noodles with Pesto and Grilled Chicken
3. Sides
   - Cauliflower Rice Stir-Fry
   - Garlic Roasted Broccoli
   - Creamed Spinach
4. Desserts

- Keto Chocolate Mousse
- Almond Flour Shortbread Cookies
- Berry Cheesecake Bars

Appetizers

Recipe 1: Garlic Butter Shrimp

Ingredients:
- 1 lb large shrimp, peeled and deveined
- 3 tbsp butter
- 4 cloves garlic, minced
- 1 tbsp lemon juice
- 1 tbsp chopped parsley
- Salt and pepper to taste

Method of Cooking:
1. Heat the butter in a large skillet over medium heat.
2. Add the garlic and cook until fragrant, about 1 minute.
3. Add the shrimp to the skillet and cook until pink and opaque, about 2–3 minutes per side.
4. Stir in lemon juice and parsley, then season with salt and pepper.
5. Serve immediately.

Cooking Time:

- Total: 10 minutes

Nutritional Information (per serving):
- Calories: 200
- Protein: 23g
- Fat: 12g
- Carbohydrates: 2g
- Fiber: 0g
- Net Carbs: 2g

Recipe 2: Caprese Salad
Ingredients:
- 2 large tomatoes, sliced
- 8 oz fresh mozzarella, sliced
- 1/4 cup fresh basil leaves
- 2 tbsp extra-virgin olive oil
- 1 tbsp balsamic vinegar
- Salt and pepper to taste

Method of Cooking:
1. Arrange the tomato and mozzarella slices on a platter, alternating between them.
2. Tuck basil leaves in between the tomato and mozzarella slices.
3. Drizzle with olive oil and balsamic vinegar.
4. Season with salt and pepper.
5. Serve immediately.

Cooking Time:
- Total: 10 minutes

Nutritional Information (per serving):
- Calories: 180
- Protein: 8g
- Fat: 14g
- Carbohydrates: 6g
- Fiber: 1g
- Net Carbs: 5g

Recipe 3: Avocado Deviled Eggs

Ingredients:
- 6 large eggs, hard-boiled and peeled
- 1 ripe avocado
- 1 tbsp lime juice
- 1 tbsp mayonnaise
- 1 tsp Dijon mustard
- Salt and pepper to taste
- Paprika, for garnish

Method of Cooking:
1. Cut the eggs in half lengthwise and remove the yolks.
2. In a bowl, mash the avocado and egg yolks together.
3. Add lime juice, mayonnaise, mustard, salt, and pepper, and mix until smooth.
4. Spoon or pipe the avocado mixture back into the egg whites.
5. Sprinkle it with paprika before serving.

Cooking Time:
- Total: 20 minutes

Nutritional Information (per serving):
- Calories: 100
- Protein: 5g

- Fat: 8g
- Carbohydrates: 3g
- Fiber: 2g
- Net Carbs: 1g

Main Dishes

Recipe 4: Baked Lemon Herb Salmon

Ingredients:
- 4 salmon filets
- 2 tbsp olive oil
- 2 tbsp lemon juice
- 1 tbsp chopped fresh dill
- 1 tbsp chopped fresh parsley
- 2 cloves garlic, minced
- Salt and pepper to taste

Method of Cooking:
1. Preheat your oven to 400°F (200°C).
2. In a small bowl, whisk together the olive oil, lemon juice, dill, parsley, and garlic.
3. Place the salmon filets on a baking sheet lined with parchment paper.
4. Brush the lemon herb mixture over the salmon filets and season with salt and pepper.

5. Bake for 12-15 minutes, or until the salmon is opaque and flakes easily with a fork.
6. Serve immediately.

Cooking Time:
- Total: 20 minutes

Nutritional Information (per serving):
- Calories: 250
- Protein: 22g
- Fat: 17g
- Carbohydrates: 2g
- Fiber: 0g
- Net Carbs: 2g

Recipe 5: Chicken Alfredo Spaghetti Squash

Ingredients:
- 1 medium spaghetti squash
- 2 tbsp olive oil
- 2 chicken breasts, cooked and sliced
- 1 cup heavy cream
- 1/2 cup grated Parmesan cheese
- 2 cloves garlic, minced
- 1 tbsp chopped parsley
- Salt and pepper to taste

Method of Cooking:
1. Preheat your oven to 400°F (200°C).
2. Cut the spaghetti squash in half lengthwise and remove the seeds.
3. Brush the cut sides with olive oil and place them face down on a baking sheet.
4. Bake for 30-40 minutes, or until the squash is tender.
5. Use a fork to scrape the spaghetti-like strands from the squash.
6. In a large skillet, heat the heavy cream and garlic over medium heat.
7. Add the Parmesan cheese and stir until the sauce thickens.
8. Add the sliced chicken and spaghetti squash strands to the skillet, and toss to combine.

9. Season with salt and pepper, and sprinkle with chopped parsley before serving.

Cooking Time:
- Total: 45 minutes

Nutritional Information (per serving):
- Calories: 400
- Protein: 28g
- Fat: 30g
- Carbohydrates: 10g
- Fiber: 2g
- Net Carbs: 8g

Recipe 6: Zucchini Noodles with Pesto and Grilled Chicken

Ingredients:
- 4 medium zucchinis, spiralized
- 2 tbsp olive oil
- 2 chicken breasts, grilled and sliced
- 1/2 cup pesto sauce
- 1/4 cup grated Parmesan cheese
- Salt and pepper to taste

Method of Cooking:
1. Heat olive oil in a large skillet over medium heat.
2. Add the zucchini noodles and cook for 3-4 minutes, until just tender.
3. Add the grilled chicken slices and pesto sauce, and toss to combine.
4. Season with salt and pepper.
5. Sprinkle with Parmesan cheese before serving.

Cooking Time:
- Total: 20 minutes

Nutritional Information (per serving):
- Calories: 350
- Protein: 30g
- Fat: 24g
- Carbohydrates: 8g

- Fiber: 2g
- Net Carbs: 6g

Sides

Recipe 7: Cauliflower Rice Stir-Fry

Ingredients:
- 1 medium head cauliflower, riced
- 2 tbsp olive oil
- 1 small onion, diced
- 2 cloves garlic, minced
- 1 cup mixed vegetables (e.g., bell peppers, carrots, peas)
- 2 tbsp soy sauce
- 1 tsp sesame oil
- 2 eggs, beaten
- Salt and pepper to taste

Method of Cooking:
1. Heat olive oil in a large skillet over medium heat.
2. Add the onion and garlic, and cook until softened, about 3 minutes.
3. Add the mixed vegetables and cook until tender, about 5-7 minutes.

4. Stir in the riced cauliflower and soy sauce, and cook until the cauliflower is tender, about 5 minutes.
5. Push the mixture to one side of the skillet and pour the beaten eggs into the empty side. Scramble the eggs until fully cooked, then mix them into the cauliflower rice.
6. Drizzle with sesame oil and season with salt and pepper.
7. Serve hot.

Cooking Time:
- Total: 20 minutes

Nutritional Information (per serving):
- Calories: 180
- Protein: 8g
- Fat: 11g
- Carbohydrates: 13g
- Fiber: 4g
- Net Carbs: 9g

Recipe 8: Garlic Roasted Broccoli

Ingredients:
- 1 large head broccoli, cut into florets
- 3 tbsp olive oil
- 4 cloves garlic, minced
- 1/2 tsp red pepper flakes (optional)
- Salt and pepper to taste
- 1/4 cup grated Parmesan cheese

Method of Cooking:
1. Preheat your oven to 425°F (220°C).
2. In a large bowl, toss the broccoli florets with olive oil, garlic, red pepper flakes, salt, and pepper.
3. Spread the broccoli in a single layer on a baking sheet.
4. Roast for 20–25 minutes, until the broccoli is tender and slightly crispy.
5. Remove from the oven and sprinkle

with Parmesan cheese before serving.

Cooking Time:
- Total: 30 minutes

Nutritional Information (per serving):
- Calories: 150
- Protein: 6g

- Fat: 12g
- Carbohydrates: 8g
- Fiber: 3g
- Net Carbs: 5g

Recipe 9: Creamed Spinach

Ingredients:
- 1 lb fresh spinach
- 2 tbsp butter
- 1 small onion, finely chopped
- 2 cloves garlic, minced
- 1 cup heavy cream
- 1/4 cup grated Parmesan cheese
- Salt and pepper to taste

Method of Cooking:
1. In a large skillet, melt the butter over medium heat.
2. Add the onion and garlic, and cook until softened, about 5 minutes.
3. Add the spinach and cook until wilted, about 3-5 minutes.
4. Stir in the heavy cream and Parmesan cheese, and cook until the sauce thickens, about 5 minutes.
5. Season with salt and pepper.
6. Serve hot.

Cooking Time:
- Total: 20 minutes

Nutritional Information (per serving):

- Calories: 220
- Protein: 6g
- Fat: 19g
- Carbohydrates: 8g
- Fiber: 4g
- Net Carbs: 4g

Desserts

Recipe 10: Keto Chocolate Mousse

Ingredients:
- 1 cup heavy cream
- 2 tbsp unsweetened cocoa powder
- 2 tbsp powdered erythritol
- 1 tsp vanilla extract
- 1/4 tsp salt

Method of Cooking:
1. In a large mixing bowl, beat the heavy cream until soft peaks form.
2. Add the cocoa powder, erythritol, vanilla extract, and salt.
3. Continue to beat until stiff peaks form.
4. Spoon the mousse into serving bowls and chill for at least 1 hour before serving.

Cooking Time:
- Total: 15 minutes (plus chilling time)

Nutritional Information (per serving):
- Calories: 200
- Protein: 2g
- Fat: 20g
- Carbohydrates: 4g
- Fiber: 1g
- Net Carbs: 3g

Recipe 11: Almond Flour Shortbread Cookies

Ingredients:
- 2 cups almond flour
- 1/4 cup powdered erythritol
- 1/2 cup butter, melted
- 1 tsp vanilla extract
- 1/4 tsp salt

Method of Cooking:
1. Preheat your oven to 350°F (175°C).
2. In a mixing bowl, combine the almond flour, powdered erythritol, melted butter, vanilla extract, and salt.
3. Mix until a dough forms.
4. Roll the dough into small balls and place them on a baking sheet lined with parchment paper. Flatten each ball slightly.
5. Bake for 10–12 minutes, until the edges are golden brown.
6. Allow the cookies to cool on the baking sheet before transferring to a wire rack to cool completely.

Cooking Time:
- Total: 25 minutes

Nutritional Information (per serving):

- Calories: 150
- Protein: 3g
- Fat: 14g
- Carbohydrates: 5g
- Fiber: 2g
- Net Carbs: 3g

Recipe 12: Berry Cheesecake Bars

Ingredients:
- 1 cup almond flour
- 3 tbsp powdered erythritol
- 1/4 cup butter, melted
- 8 oz cream cheese, softened
- 1/2 cup powdered erythritol
- 1 egg
- 1 tsp vanilla extract
- 1 cup mixed berries (e.g., strawberries, blueberries, raspberries)

Method of Cooking:
1. Preheat your oven to 350°F (175°C).
2. In a mixing bowl, combine the almond flour, 3 tbsp erythritol, and melted butter. Press the mixture into the bottom of an 8x8 inch baking dish.
3. Bake the crust for 10 minutes, then remove from the oven and let cool.
4. In another mixing bowl, beat the cream cheese and 1/2 cup erythritol until smooth. Add the egg and vanilla extract, and beat until combined.
5. Spread the cream cheese mixture over the cooled crust.
6. Top with mixed berries.

7. Bake for 20-25 minutes, until the cheesecake layer is set.
8. Allow the bars to cool completely before cutting into squares and serving.

Cooking Time:
- Total: 45 minutes

Nutritional Information (per serving):
- Calories: 180
- Protein: 4g
- Fat: 16g
- Carbohydrates: 7g
- Fiber: 2g
- Net Carbs: 5g

Recipe 13: Buffalo Cauliflower Bites

Ingredients:
- 1 large head cauliflower, cut into florets
- 2 tbsp olive oil
- 1/2 cup hot sauce (such as Frank's RedHot)
- 2 tbsp melted butter
- 1 tsp garlic powder
- Salt and pepper to taste

Method of Cooking:
1. Preheat your oven to 425°F (220°C).
2. In a large bowl, toss the cauliflower florets with olive oil, garlic powder, salt, and pepper.
3. Spread the cauliflower in a single layer on a baking sheet.
4. Roast for 20-25 minutes, until tender and slightly crispy.
5. In a small bowl, mix the hot sauce and melted butter.
6. Remove the cauliflower from the oven and toss with the hot sauce mixture.
7. Serve immediately.

Cooking Time:
- Total: 30 minutes

Nutritional Information (per serving):
- Calories: 70
- Protein: 2g
- Fat: 5g
- Carbohydrates: 6g

- Fiber: 2g
- Net Carbs: 4g

Recipe 14: Avocado Tuna Salad

Ingredients:
- 2 ripe avocados, halved and pitted
- 1 can (5 oz) tuna, drained
- 1/4 cup red onion, finely chopped
- 1/4 cup celery, finely chopped
- 2 tbsp mayonnaise
- 1 tbsp lemon juice
- 1 tbsp fresh parsley, chopped
- Salt and pepper to taste

Method of Cooking:
1. Scoop out the avocado flesh, leaving a small border inside the skins, and chop it.
2. In a bowl, combine the chopped avocado, tuna, red onion, celery, mayonnaise, lemon juice, parsley, salt, and pepper.
3. Spoon the tuna salad back into the avocado halves.
4. Serve immediately.

Cooking Time:
- Total: 15 minutes

Nutritional Information (per serving):
- Calories: 220
- Protein: 12g
- Fat: 18g
- Carbohydrates: 8g
- Fiber: 6g
- Net Carbs: 2g

Recipe 15: Mini Caprese Skewers

Ingredients:
- 1 pint cherry tomatoes
- 8 oz mozzarella balls (bocconcini)
- Fresh basil leaves
- 2 tbsp balsamic glaze
- 1 tbsp extra-virgin olive oil
- Salt and pepper to taste
- Toothpicks or small skewers

Method of Cooking:
1. Thread a cherry tomato, a basil leaf, and a mozzarella ball onto each toothpick or skewer.
2. Arrange the skewers on a serving platter.
3. Drizzle with balsamic glaze and olive oil.
4. Season with salt and pepper.
5. Serve immediately.

Cooking Time:
- Total: 15 minutes

Nutritional Information (per serving):
- Calories: 90
- Protein: 4g
- Fat: 7g
- Carbohydrates: 3g
- Fiber: 0g
- Net Carbs: 3g

Main Dishes

Recipe 16: Beef and Broccoli Stir-Fry

Ingredients:
- 1 lb beef sirloin, thinly sliced
- 4 cups broccoli florets
- 2 tbsp coconut oil
- 3 cloves garlic, minced
- 1/4 cup soy sauce or tamari
- 1 tbsp grated ginger
- 1 tbsp sesame oil
- 1 tbsp sesame seeds
- Salt and pepper to taste

Method of Cooking:
1. Heat the coconut oil in a large skillet over medium-high heat.
2. Add the beef and cook until browned, about 3-4 minutes per side.
3. Remove the beef from the skillet and set aside.
4. Add the broccoli and garlic to the skillet and cook until tender, about 5-7 minutes.
5. Return the beef to the skillet and stir in the soy sauce, ginger, and sesame oil.
6. Cook for another 2-3 minutes, until everything is well combined and heated through.
7. Sprinkle with sesame seeds before serving.

Cooking Time:

- Total: 20 minutes

Nutritional Information (per serving):
- Calories: 300
- Protein: 25g
- Fat: 18g
- Carbohydrates: 10g
- Fiber: 3g
- Net Carbs: 7g

Recipe 17: Keto Chicken Parmesan

Ingredients:
- 4 chicken breasts
- 1 cup almond flour
- 1/2 cup grated Parmesan cheese
- 1 tsp Italian seasoning
- 1/2 tsp garlic powder
- 2 eggs, beaten
- 1 cup marinara sauce (no sugar added)
- 1 cup shredded mozzarella cheese
- 2 tbsp olive oil
- Salt and pepper to taste

Method of Cooking:
1. Preheat your oven to 375°F (190°C).
2. In a bowl, mix the almond flour, Parmesan cheese, Italian seasoning, garlic powder, salt, and pepper.
3. Dip each chicken breast in the beaten eggs, then coat with the almond flour mixture.
4. Heat the olive oil in a large skillet over medium heat.
5. Cook the chicken breasts until golden brown, about 3-4 minutes per side.
6. Transfer the chicken to a baking dish.
7. Top each chicken breast with marinara sauce and mozzarella cheese.
8. Bake for 20-25 minutes, until the chicken is cooked through and the cheese is melted and bubbly.
9. Serve hot.

Cooking Time:

- Total: 35 minutes

Nutritional Information (per serving):
- Calories: 450
- Protein: 40g
- Fat: 25g
- Carbohydrates: 8g
- Fiber: 3g
- Net Carbs: 5g

Recipe 18: Zoodles with Meatballs

Ingredients:
- 4 medium zucchinis, spiralized
- 1 lb ground beef
- 1/4 cup grated Parmesan cheese
- 1/4 cup almond flour
- 1 egg
- 2 cloves garlic, minced
- 1 tsp Italian seasoning
- 2 cups marinara sauce (no sugar added)
- 2 tbsp olive oil
- Salt and pepper to taste

Method of Cooking:
1. In a bowl, mix the ground beef, Parmesan cheese, almond flour, egg, garlic, Italian seasoning, salt, and pepper.
2. Form the mixture into small meatballs.
3. Heat the olive oil in a large skillet over medium heat.
4. Cook the meatballs until browned and cooked through, about 8-10 minutes.
5. Remove the meatballs from the skillet and set aside.
6. Add the zucchini noodles to the skillet and cook until just tender, about 3-4 minutes.
7. Return the meatballs to the skillet and add the marinara sauce.
8. Cook for another 2-3 minutes, until everything is well combined and heated through.
9. Serve hot.

Cooking Time:
- Total: 25 minutes

Nutritional Information (per serving):
- Calories: 350
- Protein: 25g
- Fat: 20g
- Carbohydrates: 10g
- Fiber: 3g
- Net Carbs: 7g

Sides

Recipe 19: Bacon-Wrapped Asparagus

Ingredients:
- 1 bunch asparagus, trimmed
- 8 slices bacon
- 1 tbsp olive oil
- Salt and pepper to taste

Method of Cooking:
1. Preheat your oven to 400°F (200°C).
2. Wrap each asparagus spear with a slice of bacon.
3. Arrange the bacon-wrapped asparagus on a baking sheet.
4. Drizzle with olive oil and season with salt and pepper.
5. Bake for 15-20 minutes, until the bacon is crispy and the asparagus is tender.

6. Serve hot.

Cooking Time:
- Total: 25 minutes

Nutritional Information (per serving):
- Calories: 120
- Protein: 5g
- Fat: 10g
- Carbohydrates: 4g
- Fiber: 2g
- Net Carbs: 2g

Recipe 20: Cheesy Cauliflower Mash

Ingredients:
- 1 large head cauliflower, cut into florets
- 1/4 cup heavy cream
- 1/4 cup grated cheddar cheese
- 2 tbsp butter
- 2 cloves garlic, minced
- Salt and pepper to taste

Method of Cooking:
1. Bring a large pot of water to a boil.
2. Add the cauliflower florets and cook until tender, about 10-12 minutes.
3. Drain the cauliflower and return to the pot.
4. Add the heavy cream, cheddar cheese, butter, garlic, salt, and pepper.
5. Use a hand mixer or immersion blender to blend until smooth.
6. Serve hot.

Cooking Time:
- Total: 20 minutes

Nutritional Information (per serving):
- Calories: 150
- Protein: 5g
- Fat: 12g
- Carbohydrates: 8g
- Fiber: 3g
- Net Carbs: 5g

Recipe 21: Garlic Butter Green Beans

Ingredients:
- 1 lb green beans, trimmed
- 3 tbsp butter
- 3 cloves garlic, minced
- 1 tbsp lemon juice
- Salt and pepper to taste

Method of Cooking:
1. Bring a large pot of salted water to a boil.
2. Add the green beans and cook until tender-crisp, about 3-4 minutes.
3. Drain the green beans and set aside.
4. In a large skillet, melt the butter over medium heat.
5. Add the garlic and cook until fragrant, about 1 minute.
6. Add the green beans and toss to coat in the garlic butter.
7. Drizzle with lemon juice and season with salt and pepper.
8. Serve hot.

Cooking Time:
- Total: 10 minutes

Nutritional Information (per serving):
- Calories: 100
- Protein: 2g
- Fat: 8g
- Carbohydrates: 6g
- Fiber: 3g
- Net Carbs: 3g

Recipe 22: Roasted Brussels Sprouts with Bacon

Ingredients:
- 1 lb Brussels sprouts, halved
- 4 slices bacon, chopped
- 2 tbsp olive oil
- Salt and pepper to taste

Method of Cooking:
1. Preheat your oven to 400°F (200°C).
2. Toss the Brussels sprouts with olive oil, salt, and pepper.
3. Spread the Brussels sprouts on a baking sheet and sprinkle with chopped bacon.
4. Roast for 20-25 minutes, until the Brussels sprouts are tender and caramelized and the bacon is crispy.
5. Serve hot.

Cooking Time:
- Total: 30 minutes

Nutritional Information (per serving):
- Calories: 150
- Protein: 5g
- Fat: 12g
- Carbohydrates: 8g
- Fiber: 4g
- Net Carbs: 4g

Recipe 23: Cauliflower Fried Rice

Ingredients:
- 1 large head cauliflower, riced
- 2 tbsp coconut oil
- 1 small onion, diced
- 2 cloves garlic, minced
- 1 cup mixed vegetables (carrots, peas, bell peppers)
- 2 eggs, beaten
- 3 tbsp soy sauce or tamari
- 1 tsp sesame oil
- 2 green onions, sliced

Method of Cooking:
1. Heat the coconut oil in a large skillet over medium-high heat.
2. Add the onion and garlic, and cook until softened, about 3-4 minutes.
3. Add the mixed vegetables and cook until tender, about 5-7 minutes.
4. Push the vegetables to one side of the skillet and pour the beaten eggs on the other side.
5. Scramble the eggs until cooked through, then mix them with the vegetables.
6. Add the riced cauliflower and cook until tender, about 5 minutes.
7. Stir in the soy sauce, sesame oil, and green onions.
8. Serve hot.

Cooking Time:
- Total: 20 minutes

Nutritional Information (per serving):
- Calories: 150
- Protein: 5g
- Fat: 10g
- Carbohydrates: 10g
- Fiber: 4g
- Net Carbs: 6g

Desserts

Recipe 24: Keto Peanut Butter Cookies

Ingredients:
- 1 cup creamy peanut butter
- 1/2 cup powdered erythritol
- 1 egg
- 1 tsp vanilla extract

Method of Cooking:
1. Preheat your oven to 350°F (175°C).
2. In a mixing bowl, combine the peanut butter, powdered erythritol, egg, and vanilla extract until well mixed.
3. Roll the dough into small balls and place them on a baking sheet lined with parchment paper. Flatten each ball with a fork, making a crisscross pattern.

4. Bake for 10-12 minutes, until the edges are golden brown.

5. Allow the cookies to cool on the baking sheet before transferring to a wire rack to cool completely.

Cooking Time:
- Total: 20 minutes

Nutritional Information (per serving):
- Calories: 100
- Protein: 4g
- Fat: 8g
- Carbohydrates: 4g
- Fiber: 2g
- Net Carbs: 2g

Recipe 25: Coconut Flour Brownies

Ingredients:
- 1/2 cup coconut flour
- 1/2 cup unsweetened cocoa powder
- 1/2 cup powdered erythritol
- 1/2 cup melted coconut oil
- 4 eggs
- 1 tsp vanilla extract
- 1/4 tsp salt

Method of Cooking:
1. Preheat your oven to 350°F (175°C).
2. In a mixing bowl, combine the coconut flour, cocoa powder, powdered erythritol, melted coconut oil, eggs, vanilla extract, and salt until smooth.
3. Pour the batter into an 8x8 inch baking dish lined with parchment paper.
4. Bake for 20-25 minutes, until a toothpick inserted into the center comes out clean.
5. Allow the brownies to cool before cutting into squares and serving.

Cooking Time:
- Total: 30 minutes

Nutritional Information (per serving):
- Calories: 120
- Protein: 3g
- Fat: 9g
- Carbohydrates: 7g

- Fiber: 4g
- Net Carbs: 3g

Recipe 26: Lemon Cheesecake Fat Bombs

Ingredients:
- 8 oz cream cheese, softened
- 1/4 cup butter, softened
- 1/4 cup powdered erythritol
- 1 tbsp lemon juice
- 1 tsp lemon zest

Method of Cooking:
1. In a mixing bowl, combine the cream cheese, butter, powdered erythritol, lemon juice, and lemon zest until smooth.
2. Scoop the mixture into small balls and place them on a baking sheet lined with parchment paper.
3. Freeze for at least 1 hour before serving.

Cooking Time:
- Total: 10 minutes (plus freezing time)

Nutritional Information (per serving):
- Calories: 100
- Protein: 1g
- Fat: 10g
- Carbohydrates: 1g
- Fiber: 0g
- Net Carbs: 1g

Appetizers

Recipe 27: Jalapeno Popper Dip

Ingredients:
- 8 oz cream cheese, softened
- 1/2 cup mayonnaise
- 1/2 cup shredded cheddar cheese
- 1/2 cup shredded mozzarella cheese
- 1/4 cup diced jalapenos (fresh or pickled)
- 1/4 cup grated Parmesan cheese
- 1/4 cup pork rind crumbs

Method of Cooking:
1. Preheat your oven to 375°F (190°C).
2. In a mixing bowl, combine the cream cheese, mayonnaise, cheddar cheese, mozzarella cheese, and diced jalapenos until well mixed.
3. Spread the mixture into a baking dish.
4. In a small bowl, mix the Parmesan cheese and pork rind crumbs, then sprinkle over the dip.
5. Bake for 20-25 minutes, until the dip is hot and bubbly and the topping is golden brown.
6. Serve hot with low-carb crackers or vegetables.

Cooking Time:
- Total: 30 minutes

Nutritional Information (per serving):
- Calories: 150

- Protein: 5g
- Fat: 14g
- Carbohydrates: 2g
- Fiber: 0g
- Net Carbs: 2g

Recipe 28: Prosciutto-Wrapped Melon

Ingredients:
- 1 small cantaloupe or honeydew melon, peeled and cut into wedges
- 12 slices prosciutto
- Fresh basil leaves (optional)

Method of Cooking:
1. Wrap each melon wedge with a slice of prosciutto.
2. Arrange the wrapped melon on a serving platter.
3. Garnish with fresh basil leaves, if desired.
4. Serve immediately.

Cooking Time:
- Total: 10 minutes

Nutritional Information (per serving):
- Calories: 60
- Protein: 4g
- Fat: 3g
- Carbohydrates: 5g
- Fiber: 1g
- Net Carbs: 4g

Recipe 29: Spaghetti Squash Carbonara

Method of Cooking
6. In a bowl, whisk together the eggs, Parmesan cheese, and heavy cream.
7. Once the spaghetti squash is cooked, use a fork to scrape out the strands of squash into a large bowl.
8. Add the egg mixture to the hot squash strands and toss quickly to create a creamy sauce.
9. Stir in the cooked bacon and garlic.
10. Season with salt and pepper to taste.
11. Serve immediately.

Cooking Time:
- Total: 50 minutes

Nutritional Information (per serving):
- Calories: 250
- Protein: 12g
- Fat: 18g
- Carbohydrates: 12g
- Fiber: 3g
- Net Carbs: 9g

Recipe 30: Lemon Herb Grilled Salmon

Ingredients:
- 4 salmon filets
- 1/4 cup olive oil
- 2 tbsp lemon juice
- 2 cloves garlic, minced
- 1 tbsp fresh parsley, chopped
- 1 tbsp fresh dill, chopped
- Salt and pepper to taste

Method of Cooking:
1. In a small bowl, whisk together the olive oil, lemon juice, garlic, parsley, dill, salt, and pepper.
2. Place the salmon filets in a shallow dish and pour the marinade over them. Let marinate for at least 30 minutes.
3. Preheat your grill to medium-high heat.
4. Grill the salmon for 4-5 minutes per side, until the fish is cooked through and flakes easily with a fork.
5. Serve hot.

Cooking Time:
- Total: 40 minutes (including marinating time)
Nutritional Information (per serving):
- Calories: 350
- Protein: 34g
- Fat: 22g

- Carbohydrates: 1g
- Fiber: 0g
- Net Carbs: 1g

Sides

Recipe 31: Creamed Spinach

Ingredients:
- 1 lb fresh spinach, washed and trimmed
- 1/4 cup heavy cream
- 2 tbsp butter
- 2 cloves garlic, minced
- 1/4 cup grated Parmesan cheese
- Salt and pepper to taste

Method of Cooking:
1. In a large skillet, melt the butter over medium heat.
2. Add the garlic and cook until fragrant, about 1 minute.
3. Add the spinach and cook until wilted, about 3-4 minutes.
4. Stir in the heavy cream and Parmesan cheese.
5. Cook for another 2-3 minutes, until the mixture is thick and creamy.
6. Season with salt and pepper to taste.
7. Serve hot.

Cooking Time:
- Total: 10 minutes

Nutritional Information (per serving):
- Calories: 150
- Protein: 4g
- Fat: 14g
- Carbohydrates: 4g
- Fiber: 2g
- Net Carbs: 2g

Recipe 32: Garlic Roasted Radishes

Ingredients:
- 1 lb radishes, trimmed and halved
- 2 tbsp olive oil
- 3 cloves garlic, minced
- 1 tbsp fresh parsley, chopped
- Salt and pepper to taste

Method of Cooking:
1. Preheat your oven to 400°F (200°C).
2. In a bowl, toss the radishes with olive oil, garlic, salt, and pepper.
3. Spread the radishes on a baking sheet in a single layer.
4. Roast for 20-25 minutes, until the radishes are tender and golden brown.
5. Sprinkle with fresh parsley before serving.

Cooking Time:
- Total: 30 minutes

Nutritional Information (per serving):
- Calories: 80
- Protein: 1g
- Fat: 7g
- Carbohydrates: 4g
- Fiber: 2g
- Net Carbs: 2g

Desserts

Recipe 33: Chocolate Avocado Mousse

Ingredients:
- 2 ripe avocados
- 1/4 cup unsweetened cocoa powder
- 1/4 cup almond milk
- 1/4 cup powdered erythritol
- 1 tsp vanilla extract
- Pinch of salt

Method of Cooking:
1. In a blender or food processor, combine the avocados, cocoa powder, almond milk, powdered erythritol, vanilla extract, and salt.
2. Blend until smooth and creamy.
3. Taste and adjust sweetness if needed.
4. Chill in the refrigerator for at least 30 minutes before serving.

Cooking Time:
- Total: 10 minutes (plus chilling time)

Nutritional Information (per serving):
- Calories: 180
- Protein: 3g
- Fat: 15g
- Carbohydrates: 10g

- Fiber: 7g
- Net Carbs: 3g

Recipe 34: Keto Cheesecake Bites

Ingredients:
- 8 oz cream cheese, softened
- 1/4 cup powdered erythritol
- 1 tsp vanilla extract
- 1/4 cup almond flour
- 2 tbsp melted butter

Method of Cooking:
1. Preheat your oven to 350°F (175°C).
2. In a mixing bowl, combine the almond flour and melted butter to form a crust mixture.
3. Press the crust mixture into the bottom of a silicone mini muffin pan.
4. In another bowl, beat the cream cheese, powdered erythritol, and vanilla extract until smooth.
5. Spoon the cheesecake mixture over the crust in the muffin pan.
6. Bake for 15-18 minutes, until the cheesecake is set.
7. Allow to cool completely before removing from the pan.
8. Chill in the refrigerator before serving.

Cooking Time:
- Total: 30 minutes

Nutritional Information (per serving):
- Calories: 90
- Protein: 2g
- Fat: 8g

- Carbohydrates: 2g
- Fiber: 1g
- Net Carbs: 1g

Appetizers

Recipe 35: Deviled Eggs

Ingredients:
- 6 large eggs, hard-boiled and peeled
- 1/4 cup mayonnaise
- 1 tsp Dijon mustard
- 1 tsp apple cider vinegar
- Salt and pepper to taste
- Paprika for garnish

Method of Cooking:
1. Slice the hard-boiled eggs in half lengthwise.
2. Remove the yolks and place them in a bowl.
3. Mash the yolks with a fork and mix in the mayonnaise, Dijon mustard, apple cider vinegar, salt, and pepper until smooth.
4. Spoon or pipe the yolk mixture back into the egg whites.

5. Sprinkle it with paprika before serving.

Cooking Time:
- Total: 20 minutes

Nutritional Information (per serving):
- Calories: 60
- Protein: 3g
- Fat: 5g
- Carbohydrates: 0g
- Fiber: 0g
- Net Carbs: 0g

Main Dishes

Recipe 36: Stuffed Bell Peppers

Ingredients:
- 4 large bell peppers, tops cut off and seeds removed
- 1 lb ground beef
- 1 small onion, diced
- 2 cloves garlic, minced
- 1 cup cauliflower rice
- 1 cup shredded cheddar cheese
- 1 cup marinara sauce (no sugar added)
- 1 tsp Italian seasoning
- Salt and pepper to taste

Method of Cooking:
1. Preheat your oven to 375°F (190°C).
2. In a large skillet, cook the ground beef, onion, and garlic over medium heat until the beef is browned and the onion is softened.
3. Stir in the cauliflower rice, marinara sauce, Italian seasoning, salt, and pepper.
4. Simmer for 5-7 minutes, until the cauliflower rice is tender.
5. Remove from heat and stir in 1/2 cup of the cheddar cheese.
6. Stuff the bell peppers with the beef mixture and place them in a baking dish.
7. Sprinkle the remaining cheddar cheese on top of the peppers.

8. Cover with foil and bake for 30-35 minutes, until the peppers are tender.
9. Remove the foil and bake for an additional 5-10 minutes, until the cheese is melted and bubbly.
10. Serve hot.

Cooking Time:
- Total: 50 minutes

Nutritional Information (per serving):
- Calories: 350
- Protein: 25g
- Fat: 20g
- Carbohydrates: 12g
- Fiber: 4g
- Net Carbs: 8g

Recipe 37: Cheddar Cauliflower Tots

Method of Cooking (continued):
2. onion powder, salt, and pepper until well mixed.
3. Scoop about 1 tablespoon of the mixture and form it into a tot shape. Place the tots on a baking sheet lined with parchment paper.
4. Bake for 20-25 minutes, turning halfway through, until the tots are golden brown and crispy.
5. Serve hot wlth your favorite dipping sauce.

Cooking Time:
- Total: 35 minutes

Nutritional Information (per serving):
- Calories: 100
- Protein: 6g
- Fat: 7g
- Carbohydrates: 4g
- Fiber: 2g
- Net Carbs: 2g

Desserts

Recipe 38: Almond Flour Pancakes

Ingredients:
- 1 cup almond flour
- 2 eggs
- 1/4 cup unsweetened almond milk
- 1 tbsp coconut oil, melted
- 1 tsp baking powder
- 1 tsp vanilla extract
- Pinch of salt

Method of Cooking:
1. In a mixing bowl, whisk together the almond flour, eggs, almond milk, coconut oil, baking powder, vanilla extract, and salt until smooth.
2. Heat a non-stick skillet over medium heat and lightly grease with coconut oil.
3. Pour 1/4 cup of batter onto the skillet for each pancake.
4. Cook until bubbles form on the surface, then flip and cook until golden brown on both sides, about 2-3 minutes per side.
5. Serve hot with butter and sugar-free syrup.

Cooking Time:
- Total: 20 minutes

Nutritional Information (per serving):
- Calories: 150
- Protein: 6g
- Fat: 12g
- Carbohydrates: 5g
- Fiber: 3g
- Net Carbs: 2g

Recipe 39: Keto Chocolate Chip Cookies

Ingredients:
- 1 1/4 cups almond flour
- 1/4 cup powdered erythritol
- 1/4 cup butter, melted
- 1 egg
- 1 tsp vanilla extract
- 1/2 tsp baking powder
- 1/4 tsp salt
- 1/2 cup sugar-free chocolate chips

Method of Cooking:
1. Preheat your oven to 350°F (175°C).
2. In a mixing bowl, combine the almond flour, powdered erythritol, melted butter, egg, vanilla extract, baking powder, and salt until well mixed.
3. Fold in the sugar-free chocolate chips.
4. Scoop tablespoon-sized balls of dough onto a baking sheet lined with parchment paper.
5. Flatten each ball slightly with your hand.
6. Bake for 10-12 minutes, until the edges are golden brown.
7. Allow the cookies to cool on the baking sheet before transferring to a wire rack to cool completely.

Cooking Time:
- Total: 20 minutes

Nutritional Information (per serving):
- Calories: 100

- Protein: 3g
- Fat: 9g
- Carbohydrates: 4g
- Fiber: 2g
- Net Carbs: 2g

Appetizers

Recipe 40: Cucumber Dill Bites

Ingredients:
- 1 large cucumber, sliced into rounds
- 1/2 cup cream cheese, softened
- 1 tbsp fresh dill, chopped
- 1 clove garlic, minced
- Salt and pepper to taste

Method of Cooking:
1. In a bowl, mix the cream cheese, dill, garlic, salt, and pepper until smooth.
2. Spread a small amount of the cream cheese mixture on each cucumber slice.
3. Arrange the cucumber bites on a serving platter.
4. Garnish with additional dill if desired.
5. Serve immediately.

Cooking Time:
- Total: 10 minutes

Nutritional Information (per serving):
- Calories: 50
- Protein: 1g
- Fat: 4g
- Carbohydrates: 2g
- Fiber: 1g
- Net Carbs: 1g

Main Dishes

Recipe 41: Chicken Alfredo Spaghetti Squash

Ingredients:
- 1 large spaghetti squash
- 2 cups cooked chicken breast, shredded
- 1 cup heavy cream
- 1/2 cup grated Parmesan cheese
- 2 cloves garlic, minced
- 1 tbsp butter
- 1/4 tsp nutmeg
- Salt and pepper to taste
- Fresh parsley, chopped (for garnish)

Method of Cooking:
1. Preheat your oven to 400°F (200°C).

2. Cut the spaghetti squash in half lengthwise and scoop out the seeds.
3. Place the squash halves cut side down on a baking sheet and bake for 40-45 minutes, until tender.
4. In a large skillet, melt the butter over medium heat.
5. Add the garlic and cook until fragrant, about 1 minute.
6. Stir in the heavy cream, Parmesan cheese, nutmeg, salt, and pepper.
7. Cook until the sauce thickens, about 5-7 minutes.
8. Add the shredded chicken to the sauce and cook until heated through.
9. Once the spaghetti squash is cooked, use a fork to scrape out the strands of squash into a large bowl.
10. Pour the Alfredo sauce over the spaghetti squash and toss to combine.
11. Garnish with fresh parsley before serving.

Cooking Time:
- Total: 50 minutes

Nutritional Information (per serving):
- Calories: 400
- Protein: 28g
- Fat: 28g
- Carbohydrates: 10g
- Fiber: 3g
- Net Carbs: 7g

Sides

Recipe 42: Parmesan Roasted Asparagus

Ingredients:
- 1 lb asparagus, trimmed
- 2 tbsp olive oil
- 1/4 cup grated Parmesan cheese
- 2 cloves garlic, minced
- Salt and pepper to taste

Method of Cooking:
1. Preheat your oven to 400°F (200°C).
2. In a bowl, toss the asparagus with olive oil, garlic, salt, and pepper.
3. Spread the asparagus on a baking sheet in a single layer.
4. Sprinkle with grated Parmesan cheese.
5. Roast for 15-20 minutes, until the asparagus is tender and the cheese is golden brown.
6. Serve hot.

Cooking Time:
- Total: 25 minutes

Nutritional Information (per serving):
- Calories: 100
- Protein: 4g
- Fat: 7g

- Carbohydrates: 5g
- Fiber: 2g
- Net Carbs: 3g

Recipe 43: Zucchini Fritters

Ingredients:
- 2 medium zucchinis, grated
- 1/4 cup almond flour
- 1/4 cup grated Parmesan cheese
- 1 egg, beaten
- 2 cloves garlic, minced
- Salt and pepper to taste
- 2 tbsp olive oil

Method of Cooking:
1. Place the grated zucchini in a clean kitchen towel and squeeze out as much moisture as possible.
2. In a bowl, combine the grated zucchini, almond flour, Parmesan cheese, egg, garlic, salt, and pepper until well mixed.
3. Heat the olive oil in a large skillet over medium-high heat.
4. Scoop about 2 tablespoons of the zucchini mixture for each fritter and drop into the skillet. Flatten slightly with a spatula.
5. Cook for 3-4 minutes per side, until golden brown and crispy.
6. Drain on paper towels and serve hot.

Cooking Time:
- Total: 20 minutes

Nutritional Information (per serving):
- Calories: 90

- Protein: 3g
- Fat: 7g
- Carbohydrates: 4g
- Fiber: 2g
- Net Carbs: 2g

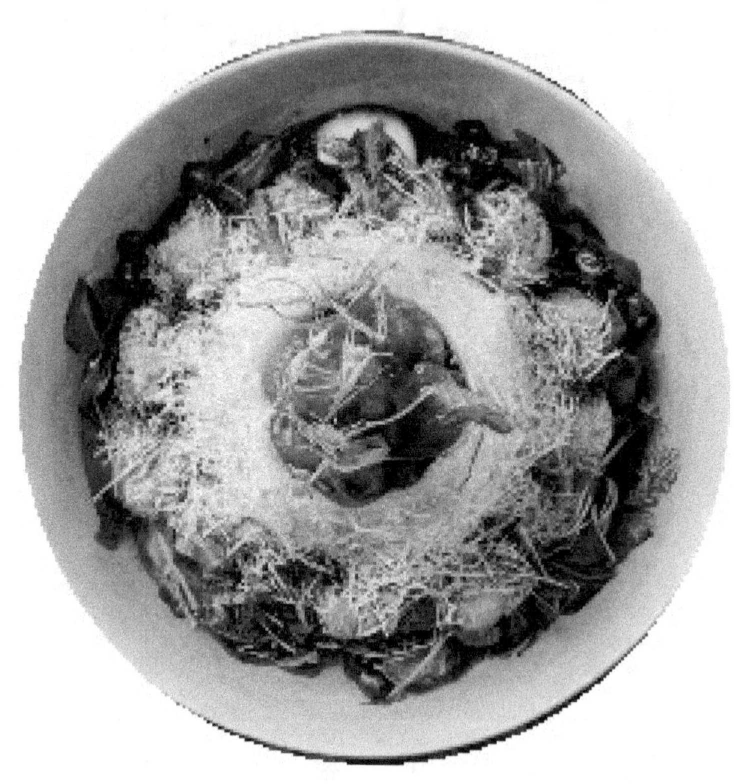

Chapter 10

The AIP diet can be adapted for vegetarians and vegans with some adjustments:

Protein Sources

- Tofu, tempeh, edamame, beans/legumes become primary protein options once reintroduced.

- Nuts, nut butters, seeds and their butters also provide plant-based protein.

- Spirulina and nutritional yeast add protein boosts to dishes.

Meal Examples

- Tofu scramble with sweet potato and spinach is a satisfying breakfast.

- Lentil sloppy joes or chili made with coconut milk instead of beef is hearty.

- Buddha bowls built with grains, beans, roasted vegetables, and avocado are filled.

- Soups, stews and curries with an assortment of veggies and proteins are balanced.

Nutrient Considerations

- B12 supplement is critical for vegans to prevent deficiency.

- Calcium from foods like kale, collards and fortified plant milks aids bone health.

- Omega-3 intake through flax, chia, walnut and seed butters is important.

- Track protein and iron needs carefully without meat to ensure adequate levels.

Sample Day
- Oatmeal with berries, nut butter
- Lentil salad bowl with roasted cauliflower
- Black bean chili with brown rice
- Trail mix
- Chia pudding

Chapter 11

Here are some quick and convenient meal ideas for busy AIP lifestyles:

- Pre-cooked rotisserie chicken: Shred for salads, sandwiches or enchiladas

- Hard boiled eggs: Easy protein for salads or snacks

- Canned salmon or sardines: Packed with omega-3s, versatile topping

- Bone broth: Heat in a mug for a warm, nourishing beverage

- AIP jerky: Store compliant meat snacks for hunger emergencies

- Frozen vegetables: Steam in the bag for an instant nutrient-dense side

- Canned coconut milk: Versatile for curries, soups, sauces or yogurt

- Pre-washed greens: Ready-to-eat salads blend on the go

- Avocado toast: Mash on cassava bread or slices of fruit for a handheld meal

- Veggie tray with nut butter: Dip raw veggies for crunch between tasks

- Smoothie pouches: Blend protein, fiber and fruits for quick hydration

- Soups/stews: Make large batches for lunches, dinners or leftover nights

- Baked potatoes/sweet potatoes: Microwave half and top as needed

With some prep on the weekends, AIP can easily accommodate busy schedules. Focus on nutrient-dense whole foods that require minimal preparation.

Chapter 12

Here are some suggestions for incorporating AIP into family meals:

- Make one main dish everyone can eat. Customize sides as needed (e.g. potatoes for non-AIP).

- Involve kids in meal prep with age-appropriate tasks like mixing, ripping lettuce, and mashing avocado.

- Present AIP meals attractively so they still look indulgent. Kids are less picky about food appearance.

- Allow "AIP nights" where the whole family follows protocol for support and learning opportunities.

- Compromise on homemade pizza/pasta night. Make AIP crust/noodles for those who need it.

- Have open communication so non-AIP family members understand restrictions without resentment.

- Keep nutritious AIP-friendly snacks visible so kids don't graze on non-compliant foods.

- Meals plan weekly family meals together so there's buy-in from all. Rotate new recipe ideas.

- Consider having AIP followers fix their own plate separately if sharing from communal dishes.

- Offer to pack an AIP-modified lunch box/bag if eating outside the home often.

- Set a good example by making AIP lifestyle seem positive, not deprived. Kids follow their parents' lead.

With creativity and teamwork, it's entirely possible for entire families to satisfy dietary needs together at mealtime.

Chapter 13

Here are some tips for using the AIP diet effectively for healthy weight management:

- Focus on whole foods. AIP emphasizes nutrient-dense choices that keep you full for long periods.

- Mind your portions. Even nutritious foods can cause weight gain if over consumed. Stop eating when satiated.

- Drink water. Stay hydrated and avoid caloric drinks which are easy to overconsume.

- Cook at home. Prepared and packaged convenience foods often have added oils, sugars and calories.

- Eat slowly. It takes 20 minutes for the stomach to signal fullness to the brain. Chew food well and be present during meals.

- Get enough protein and fat. These macronutrients promote feeling full more so than carbs.

- Track intake if needed. Weighing and measuring can raise awareness of true portions consumed.

- Manage stress. Cortisol induced by stress drives abdominal weight gain. Find relaxing activities.

- Move your body daily. Aim for 150 minutes of activity per week. Go for walks while socializing on the phone.

- Celebrate non-food victories. Praise yourself for mindfulness around lifestyle habits, not just the number on the scale.

Weight loss on AIP is gradual and sustainable when lifestyle habits support metabolic health versus quick fixes. Consistency is key.

Chapter 14

The gut-brain connection plays a key role in mental well-being. Here are some ways the AIP diet can support mood and mental health:

- Eliminates inflammatory foods like gluten and dairy which are linked to depression, anxiety, brain fog.

- Heals the gut lining to reduce absorption of toxins that can negatively impact neurotransmitters.

- Increases nutrient absorption to ensure an adequate supply of B vitamins, magnesium, omega-3s which support brain function.

-PRIORITIZES prebiotic foods like vegetables, fruits and fiber to nourish beneficial gut bacteria. This impacts serotonin and GABA levels.

- Includes plenty of anti-inflammatory foods like turmeric, ginger, berries which fight depression and boost brain health.

-Aims to remove triggers for post-ingestive distress which divert focus from living fully in the present moment.

-Encourages taking time to cook and eat meals which fosters mindfulness versus rushing or multi-tasking.

-Focuses on connecting with others while sharing meals to combat loneliness impacting mental wellness.

-Supports stabilizing blood sugar levels rather than crashing which leads to irritability and poor concentration.

Making lifestyle choices rooted in self-care like following AIP can have far-reaching benefits beyond physical health alone.

Chapter 15

Here are some ways the AIP diet supports long-term health and sustainability:

- Eliminates highly processed foods lacking nutrition. AIP prioritizes whole foods with antioxidants and phytonutrients that protect cells and reduce chronic disease risk.

- Improves gut health which is linked to longevity. The gut microbiome influences inflammation, the immune system, hormone and neurotransmitter regulation.

- Optimizes nutrient absorption to ward off deficiencies tied to accelerated aging and age-related illnesses like Alzheimer's and heart disease.

- Minimizes toxins from food sensitivities that burden the liver and produce oxidative stress damage over decades.

- Focuses on healthy fats, proteins and quality carb sources that support energy, metabolism and help maintain muscle mass in aging.

- Encourages cooking at home which is more sustainable, economical and supports building healthy lifestyle habits.

- Nurtures a positive relationship with hunger/fullness cues that prevents obesity which shortens lifespan.

- Strengthens social connections which research reliably links to increased well-being and life expectancy.

With time, commitment and consistency, following AIP long-term can translate to feeling better, avoiding preventable diseases and optimizing quality of life into advanced age.

Chapter 16

Here are some thoughts on reflecting on an AIP diet journey and looking ahead:

- Notice how your body, energy levels, mood, digestion and symptoms have changed since starting AIP. Celebrate progress made.

- Be proud of yourself for making lifestyle adjustments that benefit your long-term health and resilience. Sticking to AIP requires commitment.

- Consider if certain improvements have been sustained even after reintroducing foods. Some positive changes may reflect underlying healing beyond just diet.

- Note any foods that were reintroduced but didn't agree with you. Remain cautious of consuming large amounts of these triggers.

- Looking ahead, focus on making AIP lifestyle patterns you can maintain long-term versus viewing it as a short-term fix. Sustainability is key.

- Connect with your medical provider to discuss lab results or other markers they've monitored during your AIP experience.

- Consider maintaining AIP principles even if gradually reintroducing some foods back in. Listen to your body's unique needs.

- Remember that relapse is natural. Be gentle with yourself if symptoms return and adjust your diet as needed without guilt.

- Continue self-care practices and stress management to support ongoing healing beyond just dietary aspects of AIP.

The journey often brings as much wisdom as the destination. Reflecting helps optimally guide your path ahead.